THE MARIN COUNTY DIET:

FEED YOUR CHILD RIGHT FROM BIRTH

▲ ▲ ▲

Albert C Goldberg, MD

Ally-Han Publishing

ISBN: **0615789293**
ISBN 13: **9780615789293**
Library of Congress Control Number: **2013910163**
LCCN Imprint Name: **Larkspur, California**

▲ ▲ ▲

PART III: RESOURCES FOR PARENTS

To My Son, Keith Goldberg

12/11/61—6/14/62

who inspired me to become a pediatrician

Marin County was ranked the healthiest county in California for the fourth consecutive year in an annual survey conducted by the University of Wisconsin Population Health Institute and the Robert Wood Johnson Foundation. In addition, Marin County was named as the # 1 most kid healthy county in the entire USA according to rankings by U.S. News & World Report in 2013.

You will find yourself returning to this book over and over again. It will help you sort through exaggerations from mainstream food industry and health food industry. But most of all, THE MARIN COUNTY DIET will help parents **Feed their Child Right from Birth. Join the ranks of the healthiest County for kids in the USA.**

THE MARIN COUNTY DIET: Feed Your Child Right from Birth is a nutrition book that contains more than nutritious soups, sandwiches, and snack recipes that kids like. I've slipped in an elementary education in nutrients–just the basics–that can help parents find their way through the thicket of good nutritional information, the hype and the misinformation that's out there. I've also included charts and specific guidelines on the nutritional needs of children at various ages. The MARIN COUNTY DIET contains everything a parent needs to know to design an optimal diet for the well child.

Although I am writing this book for children, it will surely have an effect on the eating habits and good health of adult readers. What you find out about sodium, for instance, whether or not you're a parent and no matter what your age or family medical history, I believe you'll be grateful for my Five-Step Program in PART I for cutting down the amount of sodium in your food. It is important to make changes in manageable steps, and come up with foods that children will accept and incorporate into their diets.

There is a special need for a practical nutrition book that contains evidence based information rather than faith based thinking passed off as "science." Much of our nutritional information is not evidence based. It is what we were taught by our parents, grandparents, health food store salespersons, and professors at medical school. This is what I mean by "Faith Based." In addition, there are many dietary laws drawn from religions that are blindly followed by orthodox members. When possible, I will attempt to let you know when my nutritional recommendations are speculative, religion based, or what my grandmother taught me.

This, along with suggestions that a busy parent can follow, make **THE MARIN COUNTY DIET: Feed Your Child Right from Birth** such a book. To my knowledge, this is the only book that addresses the daily nutritional health issues of children in a specific, scientific and friendly way. It is not a "diet book" such as a "weight loss" book. This is my attempt to help you prevent the onset of child obesity, early cardiovascular disease, metabolic syndrome, diabetes and those illness referred to as diseases of aging. What makes pediatrics different from other branches of medicine is that the pediatrician's duty is to promote prevention, while most other medical practitioners attempt to control or treat illness after the genie escapes from the bottle. Pediatricians are in a unique position. We attend to children RIGHT FROM BIRTH.

In addition to parents, this book will be of special interest to nursery schools, elementary and high school teachers, coaches, all health care providers, family physicians, pediatricians, and nurses who work with children, including pediatric and family nurse practitioners. One of the most important duties of health practitioners is teaching families what they can do to prevent future health related illness. Most of the nutritional guides available to family practitioners bypass the special nutritional needs of children. Of those books designed for children, the recommended foods, meals, soups and sandwiches not only conflict with scientific nutritional information, but often promote foods shown to be poor nutritional choices. For example, the high fat, salt, and sugar peanut butter and jelly sandwich seems to appear alongside the high salt canned soups as a recommended food choice in most children's nutrition guides.

Many readers will not read this books straight through; therefore I have repeated important points in different sections of this book. These repetitions are deliberate to make certain that the reader who reads a book from back to front, as I often do, does not miss this information.

There are other types of nutrition books available to health educators and families and are promoted by the "Health Food " industry. These books contain the most misleading information imaginable. They put the fear of God into anyone who buys mainstream foods. They claim that high pesticide residues and poisons are around every corner, while the foods they recommend are supposed to contain exaggerated healing properties. These books are filled with claims that their recommended food choices prevent all sorts of illnesses and promote high immunity, along with other minimally substantiated information. These books state that in order to maintain optimal health one must consume multiple supplements (purchased in "Health Food Stores" and abundantly over the Internet) to counteract all our environmental toxins and boost immunity. Our U.S. Constitution gives every citizen the right of freedom of speech, therefore, it is legal to write and publish any type of information, be it true or false. This disinformation is commonly sold over the Internet to those who are truly looking for good nutritional advice.

Read my comments on Ice cream in PART I. You may be surprised. Ice cream, which we all love, is commonly treated as a food rather than an extremely high fat high sugar candy, while pizza is passed off as a "nutritious" food without regard to its highly processed, excessive salt and saturated fat content.

The food industry bias dominates these books. In **THE MARIN COUNTY DIET: Feed Your Child Right from Birth** the nutritional counterparts to these snack foods are presented in PART I and again, in greater detail, in the Nutritional Facts section of PART III.

Although most of my suggestions and anecdotes come from my years of experience nurturing thousands of children (and their parents), I have recruited the experience of many other experts in nutrition. I've footnoted the sources of many statements I've made that were based on the research or experience of other investigators. This will help those readers who wish to probe deeper into clinical nutrition with a concrete starting point. With the World Wide Web at our fingertips, obtaining original articles is now much easier. But beware; the Web is also filled with highly flawed advice. Learn about the lists of reputable online sites for nutritional information. Ask your pediatrician for help. If your doctor is unfamiliar with such a list, have him consult a local Pediatric Residency Program Director. Doctors in your medical community often maintain an updated list as well. The Council Against Health Fraud operates an important website called Quackwatch (www.quackwatch.com). This is an excellent resource for parents, teachers, coaches, nurses and physicians. I deliberately omitted other websites because they may become obsolete or undependable.

Nutrition has been an area of great interest to me since medical school. I knew what a unique position I was in as a pediatrician to influence and educate patients in practical nutrition. As a college student I visited Rodale's farm in Pennsylvania and learned about his organic farming. Rachel Carson's **Silent Spring** gave me further insight into the long-term effect of what we eat. But it was after reading Nathan Pritikin's **Live Longer Now and Campbell's The China Study** that I realized how much more I needed to learn about diet and its effect on health and disease. Nutrition, as taught in medical school, was a small part of the biochemistry and physiology curriculum. I learned what was scientifically known at the time about digestion of foods, carbohydrates, fats, proteins, minerals and vitamins. These classes gave me a fundamental understanding of how our body works and the tools to understand the merits of a good diet as well as the pitfalls of fad diets.

For the past 25 years I've worked in many countries, including Argentina, China, Chile, Colombia, Ecuador, Egypt, Ethiopia, Honduras, India, Philippines, Peru, Venezuela, and Vietnam, where poverty, ignorance, social disintegration and war have contributed to nutritional diseases. In Central and South America I've seen and treated all the classical nutritional diseases including rickets, scurvy, pellagra, and kwashiorkor. In Asia, I've witnessed the nutritional changes taking place in China, the Philippines, and India with its high white rice diet associated with type 2 diabetes, and where the introduction of the Western diet has made heart disease a new leading cause of death, replacing infectious diseases in their country. I have learned from practical experience that it is not easy to alter a person's food choices. Change involves much more than presenting nutritional information or making healthier food available. There are many complex issues involved in food choice or selection, such as one's religion, cultural background, ethnicity, one's inherited temperament, and of course the availability of competing sugary or salty snacks.

In 1967, as medical director and nutritional advisor of the first Head Start Program in Marin County, California, I developed its initial medical and nutrition program. This experience taught me how diet can improve minds as well as bodies. It is unfortunate that the well-intentioned school lunch programs subsidized by the US Department of Agriculture have turned into a dumping ground of high fat, high sodium, sugary and low fiber foods.

As a father of five plus eleven grandchildren and a pediatrician in private practice in Marin Country, California for over thirty years, I've been in a good position to witness how the average American family's diet stacks up. There has been a major shift in our children's dietary habits. Fewer families eat their dinner meal together. I have found that by eating meals together as a family our children's consumption of fruits and vegetables has increased. The health advantages to children who eat daily fruits and vegetables are discussed in more detail in the chapter, Foods Children Need-Part I.

At the turn of the century, malnutrition—the lack of certain nutrients, vitamins and minerals—was a problem second only to infection in this country and much of the world. The dietician or nutritionist was called upon to assist physicians in the dietary control of diseases after they had already developed to an advanced stage. Today malnutrition is more likely to be a case of **over consumption** of certain nutrients. Too much has replaced too little: Too much fat, too much salt and sugar, too much ultra-processed food.

In the past, traditional nutritional advice was given to optimize a child's growth and development. It was believed that if the child was growing taller and maintaining appropriate weight, good nutrition was achieved. Sufficient dairy, eggs, poultry and meats were emphasized along with the American "four foods group" diet. Today, pediatricians know that nutrition goes far beyond these simplistic concepts.

Pediatricians also know that nutritional mistakes can have serious consequences for youngsters. Although the immediate causes of death in children are no longer due to lack of nutrients, between 30%-40% of our children are now developing obesity, type-II diabetes with blood vessel diseases that will slowly kill them. These vascular diseases begin with consumption of too much fat, too much salt, too much sugar, plus insufficient fiber and anti-oxidants from real foods.

Parents and physicians share concern over the pesticides used in growing fruit and vegetables plus the new and old additives incorporated into our convenience foods. The attentive pediatrician considers these additives not only when giving nutritional advice, but also when analyzing a child's symptoms. For example when we see a child with recurrent headaches, we are likely to consider what might be wrong with his diet along with other possibilities. Foods containing **MSG** or nitrites: hot dogs, lunchmeats, or Top Ramen soups are examples of common headache triggering foods and are discussed in greater depth in the section covering foods associated with headaches.

More and more I talk to parents about their children's healthy diet—and this is good, because consumers have become much smarter than we were a generation ago about eating properly and reading food labels. But it's difficult to keep current with all the misinformation constantly being fed to us by a self-serving food industry.

Although food labels have improved, they are of limited value for understanding children's nutritional needs and at times downright confusing even to the well educated.

For example, the current Nutrition Facts label does not differentiate between added sugar and total sugar. In orange juice how much sugar comes naturally from the fruit and how much is added sugar? There is no way of knowing from the present Nutrition Facts label.

Furthermore, new foods are regularly added to our already superfluous choices—50% of what we see on the shelves of our supermarkets didn't even exist 25 years ago. Frozen pizza and chicken nuggets, Gatorade, sports or energy bars and drinks, instant breakfasts, and of course the constant introduction of new dry cereals are all fairly new phenomena. Kids seem to prefer these foods. How do we know if they're any good or even more important, are they harmful? And what can we provide that is nutritious, easy to prepare and that the child will like? An entire section of this book, PART III, is devoted to help you make informed choices at the supermarket. Readers will find the answers to these and many other frequently asked questions about what kids should eat and don't eat.

THE MARIN COUNTY DIET: Feed Your Child Right from Birth is organized into three parts. Part I includes the nutritional needs of infants, children and adolescents. There are three chapters in Part One. I discuss the **Nutritional Needs of Infants, Children and Adolescents**, the real world of appetite and lack of appetite, of stubbornness and curiosity, of food habits good and bad, of food fads and fad diets. Each chapter in this section focuses on children of a certain age, and each spotlights foods of particular value enjoyed at that age. For instance, the chapter **Feeding Your Infant** explores the art and science of breastfeeding, formula selection, preparation, and feeding for infants from birth through the 12th month. Regular cow milk, skim milk, evaporated milk, and goat milk are not usually recommended for children under a year old. Readers find out why in this chapter.

Chapter Two continues with **First Foods**. At four to seven months, babies may require more calories than breast milk or formula provides, and parents may introduce semisolid foods. I suggest what's appropriate and what's not, unfortunately most of which is speculation. Foods that are potential allergens are flagged, and the over and under diagnosis of wheat, gluten, and milk intolerance is discussed as is the infant's special need for iron at this age. Fruits, vegetables, cereals and liquids other than milk are featured. In this chapter I show how food manufacturers subliminally suggest to parents that juices need to be introduced into an infant's diet.

Chapter Three covers the **Toddler, Preschooler, Older Child, and Adolescent Diet.** Most children begin to eat table foods between one and two years of age. Picky eating may present itself, and here is when food habits–good and bad–begin to form. The folly of giving juice, crackers, raisins and grapes—"I know it's not great food, but it's better than nothing," is explored and how this is often the first step to a poor diet. Here I offer helpful suggestions gleaned from years of experience to help parents through these difficult months. Salt and sugar are featured, along with the complex carbohydrates such as potatoes, corn, wheat, grains, legumes and crucifers, some of the basic foods that should form the heart of your youngster's expanding diet. As in all the chapters, easy to prepare recipes for dishes that your whole family will enjoy are included.

The **Pre-school** child tastes independence! You may yearn for yesterday's picky eater when your child begins demonstrating rigid preferences and prejudices toward foods that some two to six year olds do. The solutions are sometimes simple, but often not obvious.

The child is independent at this age. Parents are no longer able to control every bite the child takes and begin to worry whether he's eating enough, eating too much, or eating the right things. This chapter is big on snacks–lots of them, good ones, ones to make at home–with guaranteed-to-please recipes included. Avoid mealtime fights and stress. Mealtimes should be pleasant, and a relaxing time of day. It's a time for comparing notes with spouses and being a role model for your children. A parent's job is to buy and prepare wholesome foods. The child's job is to decide how much to eat. Don't turn into a "short-order cook" and prepare special meals for each member of the family unless you have a special needs child. Learn how to smile and say, " This is what I prepared for dinner. If you don't wish to eat it now I'll save it for you in case you get hungry later." Your child won't starve if he chooses to leave the table to play, but be sure not to let him fill up on crackers, cookies, milk, juice, raisins and bananas!

School age, **Pre-Teen**, **and Teenagers**: Your children's socialization is likely to have a profound effect on their eating habits. Your careful attention to balanced meals, nutritious snacks, conscientious shopping and all the good this has done may meet its gravest challenge during your children's school years. This chapter considers the school-agers' and teenagers' special nutritional needs, vegetarianism, the special needs of children who get into sports, how menstruation affects nutritional needs, and the special nutritional requirements of pregnant teenagers. This chapter highlights the importance of snacking and debunks the concept of three square meals. If you can make nutritious breakfasts available at home, even nutritious breakfasts that can be eaten on the fly, you go a long way toward meeting the challenge. If you can offer a nutritious box of favorite snacks to your child or teenager, this will better serve him or her than the ever-present vending machine filled with high fat, sugary granola bars, ice cream, burritos, hot dogs, chips, nachos, fruit juice, sport drinks, or the highly processed salted chicken or turkey sandwich. The anything-but-nutritious lunches most school cafeterias serve provide fertile territory for those activists who read this book and wish to make constructive suggestions to those responsible for school lunch programs. My ideas for easy-to-prepare delicious and truly nutritious lunches and suppers are also featured.

Part II takes a close look at the specific nutritional needs, likes and dislikes of children as they grow. I call this part, THE CHEMICALS OF LIFE. That sounds less threatening than BIOCHEMISTRY 101. The Chemicals of Life is a primer to help understand the basics of what infants, children and adolescents nutritional needs, and what foods will fulfill those needs. Also, I discuss foods detrimental to children's health, and how the food industry hypes its products with blatantly deceptive advertising copy and empty claims.

Part II devotes a chapter each to **Carbohydrates**, **Proteins**, **Fats**, **Fiber, Vitamins and Minerals**, –with tables in all these categories to help the reader estimate the individual nutritional needs of infants, children, teenagers, and young adults–without being a mathematical wizard. In addition, in each of these categories I offer anecdotes and reminiscences, nutritional facts and fiction, and a cornucopia of foods high in the various nutrients but low in sugar, saturated fat and salt. Among these are occasional child-tested delicacies–easy to prepare, nutritious, and delicious–to illustrate how good nutrition appears on the plate.

Part III contains NUTRITION FACTS AND RECIPIES. This section is a guide on how to read the **Nutrition Facts** as they are on food labels, and Kid-**tested Recipes. Nutrition Facts Labels** and the now outdated **Nutrition Pyramid** are explained as well as the "**Plate**" substitute. See how your choices fit your healthier way of living. Select a truly balanced diet for your child. The **Kid-tested Recipes** section is loaded with practical nutritional pearls. They include:

On-the-fly breakfast suggestions and recipes.

Nutritious snacks that can be used as a substitute for lunch or dinner.

The art of seduction: preparing meals the way children like them.

The art of compromise. (This isn't a perfect world!).

Food suggestions at the Chinese, Italian, or Mexican fast food restaurant.

Foods that should be avoided except on very special occasions

Methods on how to modify your favorite unhealthy recipe.

How to change it to a healthy one and STILL love it.

The Guide to Eating Out With Children, the Fast Food Restaurant and learning the Art of Compromise is a

fitting conclusion to my book. This section is filled with suggestions on how to deal with food choices

when eating outside the home. As a parent, I know it's neither fair nor wise to "outlaw" foods. That is

why I have devoted an entire section to help you and your child face the world of foods outside your home.

And don't forget to explore my recommended list of Internet nutrition sites.

But most of all,

Feed Your Child Right from Birth and join the ranks of the healthiest County in California.

Albert C. Goldberg, MD
Marin County
Larkspur, California

PART I

▲ ▲ ▲

THE MARIN COUNTY DIET

FEED YOUR CHILD RIGHT FROM BIRTH

FEEDING YOUR INFANT

▲ ▲ ▲

First of all, it is important for every mother to pay special attention to what she eats beginning with the first moments she becomes aware that she is pregnant, and if it is a planned pregnancy, to begin well before trying to become pregnant. The foods that a mother eats during pregnancy affect the health of the baby. That means avoiding alcoholic beverages, foods high in mercury[1] and starting a multivitamin mineral preparation containing extra iron and folic acid.

Drink sufficient water and less coffee; eat fish that is high in DHA, such as salmon; low or non fat dairy and calcium rich foods; legumes, such as black beans or kidney beans; brown rice; fruit rich in antioxidants and vitamin C such as citrus fruit, organic

---

[1] The fish that have the highest level of mercury are shark, swordfish, king mackerel and tilefish; these are fish to avoid. Check local advisories about the safety of fish caught in your local lakes, rivers, and coastal areas. Pregnant moms can consider eating fish that are generally lower in mercury. These include shrimp, canned light tuna, salmon, Pollack, catfish, sole, flounder, and red snapper.

strawberries and organic blueberries; whole grain breads and cereal; and especially leafy greens. Eat iron-rich or iron-fortified foods such as lean meats or meat alternatives.

Breastfeeding provides the best nutrition for an infant, and the practice is gaining in popularity as more information is reaching parents. Breast milk is truly a magic food, and your breast milk is unique to your baby. It is more variable and valuable than what is suggested in scientific tables found in standard nutrition books.

Diet affects the composition of breast milk. A vegetarian's breast milk is different in fatty acid pattern from that of a non-vegetarian. Breast milk also changes depending on the age of the baby–the breast milk produced by the mother of a preterm infant is more suited to the needs of her baby and is not the same as the milk from the mother of a full term infant. At nine months of age the breast fed baby is receiving milk which is different from the milk received at one week and depending on what mother eats, the milk may taste differently from day to day, compelling the infant to adapt to new tastes. This prepares your baby's palate for when you introduce semisolid foods. Milk expressed in the first few minutes of breastfeeding, called **fore milk**, has a lower fat content than **hind** or later milk. That is one important reason why many infants need to nurse longer than a few minutes at a time. One mother may nurse briefly a few times a day and the baby rapidly gains weight while another mother may have to nurse two to three times as long and more often to provide as many calories to her infant. If your infant breastfeeds less than the time "suggested" by your "how to breastfeed" books, and your baby is thriving, don't fret! Breast milk varies tremendously from mother to mother.

Breast milk is high in saturated fats and cholesterol and there is good reason for this. Many parents look at the listed ingredients on a can of infant formula and wonder why it contains so much saturated fat, cholesterol and sugar, since they have been told repeatedly that fats, cholesterol and sugar should be avoided in their diets. Babies are different. They are not merely small adults! **Babies need saturated fat, cholesterol and milk-sugar.** Ample amounts of these nutrients are essential in these early months because of the baby's high energy needs and rapid growth of the brain and nervous system. Infant nutrition becomes even more complicated, because the amount and types of unsaturated fat and fatty acids found in breast milk are different from what is found in other animal milks such as cow or goat milk. This is one of the reasons it is so important for parents to have some understanding of the more complex nutritional needs of children, and to respect the possibility that there are probably many more nutritional unknowns to be discovered.

Most parents are not aware that **infants breast fed for greater than six months may be 5 to 9 IQ points smarter than matched formula fed infants**[2]. Certain types of **fatty acids** (docosahexaenoic acid or DHA and arachidonic acid or ARA) found in breast milk may have a part in this and is now added to commercial formulas. There are intestinal maturing factors found only in breast milk and **colostrum, the first milk present at birth,** that protects the infant from food allergies and intestinal infections. This may be reason enough to try breastfeeding, even if you must stop early to return to work or for other personal reasons. Keep in mind the option of using a high quality electric breast pump to prolong breastfeeding. This will allow your baby to receive the benefits of breast milk while you are away and also give other family members added opportunities to feed and bond with the new baby.

Although breast milk contains a lot of fat, it must be absorbed by the baby to do any good. **Lipase is an enzyme which digests fat;** it comes primarily from the pancreas. At birth and for the first few weeks of life, **pancreatic lipase** is in short supply, possibly

[2] Lancet 1992-339: 261-64.

due to the immaturity of the pancreas. Pancreatic lipase can't be given by mouth to correct this deficiency because it would be destroyed by the stomach acid before reaching the intestine. Breast milk contains a lipase which resists stomach acid and which aids pancreatic lipase in the digestive process. Neither cow nor goat milk contains this unique enzyme. So it is possible that this extra lipase helps breast fed infants to absorb more fat. Another lipase, called **lingual lipase,** comes from the base of the infant's tongue and is produced in response to sucking. This may help to explain why babies, particularly in the first few months of life, want to continue sucking even after they have finished breastfeeding . This **"non-nutritive sucking"** has been used as a rational justification for offering a pacifier to a newly born infant.[3]

The salt content of breast milk is only 150mg per liter, whereas cow milk contains 500mg per liter or over three times as much salt. **It is unknown whether this extra salt intake from cow milk could set a baby up for high blood pressure later in life, but this remains a worrisome consideration.** About 20% of infants are salt sensitive. This is one area of research that desperately needs to be studied by a major university, but in the meantime, with lack of scientific proof to guide us, the low salt content of breast milk should be our model. I trust nature's model better than the food industry or nutritionists who suggest salt may not be a bad addition to an infant's or child's diet!

Parents are led to believe that lots of minerals and calcium are good for young children, but cow and goat milk have a much greater mineral content than human milk, and this could harm

[3] Nursery nurses often promote the pacifier because it calms the hungry infant. It is used in the noble spirit of letting the tired or often exhausted mother get some needed rest. What is not appreciated is that as a consequence of this, the mother's breasts are not stimulated sufficiently, and as a result there is often a delay in milk production. The seemingly benign and benevolent act of giving the pacifier (or bottles of water) during the few days following birth is often responsible for "nursing failure." Please restrain from the temptation of using a pacifier until your milk production is enough for your infant to achieve adequate weight gain.

an infant. The high calcium content in cow milk, (1200mg vs. 300 mg in breast milk!) is too great a load on the infant's immature kidneys and should be avoided until the baby is over 12 months old. Most store-bought formulas contain about 500mg of calcium per liter. Another reason to avoid cow milk during the first year of life is its high phosphorus content–six times that of human milk. In rare cases, such a high phosphorus content can drop calcium levels in the blood, causing newborns to have seizures.

The iron content of breast milk may appear to be tiny at only 0.5mg per 100ml. However, almost 50% of this iron is absorbed, making it the most usable iron available. Cow milk contains nearly the same amount of iron but, by contrast, only 10% is absorbed. Infants who drink low iron cow milk often become iron deficient by 10 months! For this reason most cow milk formula is fortified with 12-18mgs of iron per liter. **Contrary to popular myth, this added iron will not lead to iron overload, bowel discomfort, spitting up, colic or constipation. Premature infants may have diminished stores of iron and iron supplementation may be recommended by your pediatrician or health provider.**

Trace elements found in breast milk are different in type and concentration compared with cow or goat milk. As an example, there is less zinc in human milk than in cow milk, but a baby can use almost 60% of it. The zinc present in cow milk, although higher in milligrams is only about 45% available for use. Adequate zinc is needed to enhance infant growth. Also, a baby who gets too little zinc may be very cranky or suffer from an eczema-like rash on hands, feet, face, and the genital region. Zinc is added to commercial formulas to correct for this deficiency.

A look at the vitamin content of breast milk and formula reveals some interesting comparisons. Both human and cow milk are rich in Vitamin A and Vitamin B Complex. Cow milk is low in Vitamin C. For this reason, babies fed cow milk alone need supplements. Well nourished mothers produce milk sufficient in Vitamin C. Cow milk has no Vitamin D. Because of this, rickets[4] was a common occurrence in the past and still is in countries where milk is not fortified with Vitamin D3. This vitamin may also be in low supply in breast milk. Vitamin supplements therefore are a good idea for babies, especially those who get little sunlight.[5]

Goat milk is low in folic acid (folate), and because of this infants fed only goat milk often develop a severe anemia called megaloblastic anemia. Goat milk has achieved fad status in some circles because of its falsely supposed likeness to breast milk. Parents who are concerned about their infant's slow weight gain, irritability, or frequent infections, are tempted to try goat milk as a remedy. But for reasons pointed out above, it is better to defer offering goat milk during the first year. Before making such a change, discuss this with your doctor.

Another vitamin that is low in human milk but needed for blood clotting, is **vitamin K. Breast fed infants are prone to a bleeding disease which in rare cases results in sometimes fatal bleeding into the brain.** Fortunately, this can be prevented by giving the infant Vitamin K, either by mouth or by shot. Vitamin K is now given by a nurse to almost all infants shortly after birth. Cow **milk formulas are fortified with extra Vitamin K so babies on formula are actually less susceptible** to this disease than those who are breastfed. The breast fed infant remains low in vitamin K the first 8 days of life. Religious Jews delay circumcising their son until he is 8 days old. This is the time it takes bacteria in the intestines to produce sufficient Vitamin K. It is this Vitamin K that is needed to prevent prolonged bleeding after circumcision.

Vitamin E is found in greater amounts in human milk than in cow milk. Skimmed cow milk contains no Vitamin E. Infants

---

4 *Rickets is a disease of children, characterized by softening of the bones as a result of lack of Vitamin D. Refer to Part II for more information on how sunshine helps the body manufacture Vitamin D.

5 There is more detailed information on vitamins in Part II. Please refer to this section.

fed only non-fat milk develop what is called **"failure to thrive,"** infections, extremely dry skin, and blood problems.

Besides the immune factors, growth, and brain development factors found in breast milk, I'm certain it contains many other yet undiscovered nutritional factors that nature created during our evolution. I strongly suggest that mothers continue to nurse for at least six months whenever possible, or better yet, up to one year.

It is the art of breastfeeding rather than the chemistry of breast milk that is of importance right away to a new mother. The nurturing aspect of has a potent emotional effect upon the bond between infant and mother. Unfortunately, there are a lot of worries around breastfeeding, and many myths exist. Therefore, the aid of a well-trained helper is the most important first step in breastfeeding. Beware of the helper who suggests pacifiers, sugar water or putting the infant on an "every 2-3 hour schedule" the first week of life. **This advice usually leads to insufficient sucking, which in turn leads to a delay in milk production, and in turn leads to a frustrated exhausted mother who turns to a formula.** At that moment the infant gobbles down the formula and the mother concludes that the infant has chosen not to breastfeed. Often, the physician agrees and thus pays only lip service to breastfeeding. There are now a group of specialist nurses, **lactation consultants**[6]**,** who truly understand the art and science of breastfeeding, and I recommend that one be consulted on the day of your infant's birth. Different opinions and techniques can be very confusing to the new mother. A breastfeeding specialist, along with your pediatrician, can help you establish a plan for the early weeks of breastfeeding that is specific to your baby's needs and breastfeeding style.

Formulas should be reserved for those who truly can't breastfeed or for those who choose not to breastfeed only after being taught about the nutritional advantages of breast milk. The final decision for or against breast-feeding should rest with the

[6] Ideally an I.B.C.L.C. (International Board Certified Lactation Consultant).

mother. In the meantime, don't think breastfeeding is another fad. It has been tested for thousands of years and has followed the evolution of our species.

Infant's sucking on a breast stimulates jaw development and therefore this should be encouraged when possible instead of putting pumped breast milk in a bottle.

When a mother doesn't want to breastfeed - or, can't, the second choice is a store bought formula of cow milk base, or sometimes an "elemental formula."[7] Ideally, your baby's doctor should prescribe the specific formula, technique of preparation, and appropriate schedule for bottle feeding. These directions should be based on your baby's own nutritional and digestive needs.

Formula hasn't always been a risk-free second choice. By ignoring the composition of breast milk as a model, company nutritionists created formulations that sickened some infants. The lesson: in determining infant formula's nutritional specifications, a formula should match as closely as possible the functional composition of human breast milk. The dictum, "eat a variety of foods," to protect against nutritional unknowns, does not hold for the infant who relies solely upon a single food (formula). There is no room for error when our children are the experimental creatures. Your pediatrician needs to be especially knowledgeable about formulas and not consider them all to be alike. The American Academy of Pediatrics and the FDA are constantly examining the make up of breast milk in order to make recommendations for reformulating commercial formulas. The Infant Formula Act of 1980 (revised in 1986) directs the FDA to ensure the safety and nutritional quality of infant formulas.

[7] An elemental formula is one which contains no whole protein, but instead has only the building blocks of protein (amino acids) that make up the bulk of the elemental formula along with carbohydrates, fats, vitamins and minerals.

Here are a few more bottle feeding tips:

1. **Select a nipple that is available in most drug stores. Infants become attached to the nipple they are started on and often refuse to use another type. I can recall horror stories from parents who were up all night going from one pharmacy to another searching for the only type nipple their infant would take.**
2. **Select a bottle that is BSA free. The plastic bag type bottles, such as Playtex, do not prevent air swallowing. Infants swallow air regardless of the bottle type and this is normal. Colic or gassiness is not prevented by this type of bottle.**
3. **Bottles do not need to be boiled or sterilized. They can be cycled through the dishwasher or washed and rinsed well by hand using a bottlebrush. Extra rinsing is important in order to remove all residual detergent.**[8]
4. **Boiling nipples will destroy them. Wash them thoroughly by hand with soap and water and allow the nipples to air dry in a clean cup or bowl.**
5. **Both glass or plastic bottles are OK as long as they do not contain BSA or other endocrine disruptors.**[9] **I prefer the plastic ones since they won't break when the baby throws one across the room.**

---

[8] Do not warm bottles in the microwave. Warming of the bottle's contents is uneven and the formula continues to cook for about a minute after removing the bottle from the microwave. An infant's tongue and mouth could easily be scalded by a bottle heated this way.

[9] Endocrine disruptors are chemicals with the potential to interfere with the function of the hormone system and can include plasticizers (BSA), pesticides (DDT), and natural chemicals found in plants (phytoestrogens).

Here are a few hints to prevent tender breasts:

1. Use a hair dryer to blow-dry your breast for about 20-30 seconds after each breastfeeding. This is very soothing and helps healing or tender breasts.

2. Be sure the infant takes more than the tip of the nipple into its mouth. Remove the infant from the breast by first breaking the suction with your finger.

3. Correct position is critical. Call a lactation specialist immediately if you even think you might be having any breastfeeding problem. Do not delay. Small problems are easier to solve than big ones.

4. Don't allow yourself to become frustrated. Some infants are not very interested in breastfeeding the first 24 - 36 hours , especially after a cesarean section. Ask your lactation helper whether an electric (Madela) breast pump is needed.

5. Fatigue and poor nutrition are enemies to good breastfeeding. Rest and good eating are essential. This is not the time to go on a crash diet. **A new mom needs a helper at home**. She doesn't need a nurse! The helper should take care of running the home, the cleaning, shopping, preparing food, laundry, and giving that two-year-old sibling some special attention. If daddy, or grandma is not an option, enlist a relative or close friend to help. If your budget can afford it, hire a helper. The feeling of isolation and facing the responsibility of running a household in addition to caring for an infant is often overwhelming and has a profoundly negative effect upon successful breast-feeding.

6. A nipple shield (Madela brand) may be needed for inverted nipples, as well as a high quality electric breast pump. Consult a lactation specialist at least one month before the delivery of your baby if you have inverted nipples or if you are not certain. There are many things that can be done early to

keep this from becoming a problem. The lactation specialist may suggest devices that can be worn under the bra and over the nipple, during the month prior to delivery. She will let you know, after examining your breasts, if you need them.

Pediatricians are often non-scientific in the manner in which they first select and later switch formulas. Since many infants are irritable or colicky beginning at two weeks of age through three-and-a-half months of life, a ritual of formula changing usually begins when the baby is about ten days old. By that time the desperate calls begin with predictable regularity. Instead of carefully explaining the nature of **colic**[10], the physician often elects to take the shortcut and **changes the formula.** This usually keeps the telephone quiet for another 2-3 days!

What happened to me when I cared for my oldest daughter is typical. At the time I was in my third year of medical school and I was about to learn my first practical lesson in pediatrics. She

---

[10] *Nobody has yet determined, with certainty, the cause of colic. This periodic fussiness appears at about two weeks of age and often persists to three and one half months. Colic peaks around six weeks of age and then gradually becomes less intense. Most infants have a daily "fussy"period between 5 p.m. and 11 p.m. During this time the infant cries, turns red in the face, draws up his or her legs, passes gas and appears to be in pain. The source of the pain is unclear, but most parents believe the pain arises in the gastrointestinal tract and therefore call it a bellyache or think it is constipation. For this reason parents blame the pain on diet, if it is a breast-fed baby, or the formula, in formula fed infants. There is little proof that milk formula, with or without iron, is the culprit. Nevertheless changing formulas is the traditional advice, if for no other reason than to "buy time" until the infant is over three months old. Than miraculously the baby is able to tolerate breast milk even if the mother eats beans, cabbage or drinks cow milk. The formula-fed infant now tolerates formulas that were stopped earlier. The scientific community doubts that allergy to milk or lactose intolerance is often the cause of this periodic fussiness or "colic." Nothing better than walking your infant during these hours has been invented, but swings, music, vibrating beds, and other devices have been helpful. Many medicines have been tried. Sometimes they seem to work, but the placebo effect may be the cause of temporary improvement. There are a host of other things that can be done to help parents through this stressful period. Be sure to let your pediatrician know if your child has symptoms of colic.

was breastfed for 4-6 weeks. In those years most infants were bottle fed. If the mother breastfed, it was rare to continue beyond three months. My daughter was a skinny and irritable infant. Her knees were always red because they were in constant motion. She cried often, starting at ten days of age, and with such persistence, at first in the middle of the night, and later beginning at 4-5p.m., that we were asked to move from our apartment because the neighbors couldn't stand the noise!

Later, even hours after breastfeeding or taking her formula, she would spit up. Our pediatrician suggested that my wife stop eating dairy, chocolate, "gassy vegetables" and spicy foods. For a couple of days we thought our daughter was improving, but by the weekend she was back at it. Like clockwork, as soon as I came home at around 5p.m. she started crying and fussing until after midnight. We were then instructed to try another formula. But our daughter continued to draw up her legs, turn red and cry, pass gas, and cry again. Next a soy formula was suggested. "This may be easier to digest," he explained. The colic continued. Another brand of soy formula was then recommended with similar disappointment. Maybe she's constipated, I reasoned. The elderly lady down the hall suggested a "suppository" or inserting the "end of a thermometer." We were willing to try almost anything and did this unhealthy maneuver for a few days. At first I thought we were on to a cure, but it soon became clear that the relief was not long lasting. "Perhaps the baby can't handle the iron in the formula," was the next week's telephoned advice. I later learned there was about as much iron in the soy formula he recommended as was in the last formula. The spitting and crying persisted after what I thought might have been a one or two day reprieve. The next suggestion seemed to help the most. Our doctor showed us how to swaddle her, and this did have some calming effect. He also suggested that we have her sleep in her infant seat to prevent "reflux," and prescribed an antacid and anti-gas drops. In those days gasoline was cheap, so I would buckle her in her car seat and drive around the block for an hour. Another popular method is to put the infant in a seat on the dryer. This motion has a calming effect. I promised the landlady I'd do this nightly, but she still asked us to leave our second apartment. We had three different apartments that first year of our daughter's life.

With all the scientific progress we have made over the past decade, no treatment surpasses holding and walking a colicky infant. There is little evidence that changing formulas or putting a breastfeeding mother on a "dairy-free, non-gassy, or non-spicy food" diet helps colic, but such advice continues to be freely prescribed. For the past few years, prescribing colicky infants anti-reflux medication had become another popular non-evidence based practice.

There are many excellent books to be found on breastfeeding, however , The Womanly Art of Breastfeeding as well as The Breastfeeding Mother's Guide to Making More Milk are highly recommended.

FIRST FOODS

Breast-fed infants who were given complementary foods at age 4 months had similar growth rates and better iron status at age 6 months than exclusively breast-fed infants, according to a study in the Journal "Pediatrics." Infant growth rate did not differ significantly between the two groups. However, infants in the complementary-food group had significantly higher iron stores than the exclusively breast-fed infants. Based on this information I usually recommend beginning complementary foods at 4-6 months.

The timing of the introduction of semi-solid foods to infants is confusing to parents and physicians alike. As a pediatrician in training I was taught to have infants avoid dairy until age 1 year, eggs until 2 years, peanuts, tree nuts, and seafood until 3 years

At 4 to 6 months, the baby may require more calories than breastfeeding provides, and you may decide to introduce semi-solid foods (Often referred to as, "Complementary" food). The bottle-fed baby may also be interested in exploring different tastes and textures. Feeding the infant may also afford the father[11] a chance to bond or fall in love with his baby. Many people believe that introducing semi-solid food at two to three months, especially at the last feeding of the evening, will cause an infant to sleep through the night. After all, it seems logical that the increase in bulk will keep the baby full longer. Unfortunately, armchair reasoning has to give way to careful studies which show that semi-solid foods in the diet have no or minimal effect on the age at which an infant begins to sleep through the night.

Because the rapidly growing infant needs iron to build muscle and red blood cells, I recommend an iron-fortified cereal such as baby brown rice and oatmeal cereal. On a practical level, these commercially available dry cereals are a convenient way to get your baby used to taking semi-solid foods by spoon. Infants fed iron-fortified commercial formula usually get sufficient iron from this source; however, iron rich foods are needed the first year and beyond to fulfill the needs of a rapidly growing infant, especially if the infant were born prematurely.

Because eating habits begin early, I strongly encourage parents to introduce nutritionally important foods early. Don't be afraid to introduce other cereals, such as barley, rye, and wheat. These are recommendations that are best described as traditional, and not evidence based. Avoid putting cereal or foods in a bottle as it delays a baby's adjustment to textures. Some parents do this and go on with chores. Instead, hold or attend your infant during feedings. Your baby needs this attention and social

---

[11] This should not be interpreted to mean that fathers need to feed their baby to fall in love with them. We know that many fathers fall in love with their baby without ever feeding them.

contact. After all, feeding an infant is more than nutrition. If you are too busy to feed food to your infant, delay the semi-solid part of the feeding until you have time to relax and nurture your baby. Enjoy the baby during this special period in his life. It goes by quickly!

Experiment with textures, first by adding breast milk or formula to the dry cereal to make a thin gruel and then gradually make it thicker if the infant tolerates it without gagging. I'm not aware of any scientific studies that examine the long term consequences of early versus later exposure to different tastes or textures. One good reason for starting semi-solids in the first place, is to give the non-breast fed baby a variety of foods as a safeguard against the nutritional unknowns.[12]

Many parents want to know exactly how many teaspoons of food to give their child and wonder how to tell whether the baby is getting enough or too much. The answers you will find in most baby books are intentionally vague. That is because babies vary so much in their specific needs. All those charts and calorie formulas are guidelines that are seldom necessary to use. Look at your child. Is he or she too thin? Then offer more food or increase the frequency of feedings. Too plump? Then decrease amounts a little. If you are uncertain, the safest thing is to discuss this important issue with your pediatrician or health provider during a "well child" checkup where the baby can be weighed, measured and observed in person.

Don't believe that a fat baby is healthier than a slender infant. Many breastfed infants are slender, and this may be normal, especially among certain ethnic groups. A fat infant may become a fat adult. If obesity runs in your family, be especially careful

[12] The caveat, "Eat a variety of foods," is difficult to follow if your only food source is breast milk. Fortunately, breast milk is a near perfect food for infants. If an infant's total diet is commercial formula, a vital nutrient may be missing. So until we learn a lot more about how to make a perfect formula, it may be wise to add a variety of semi-solid foods to an infant's diet beginning at four to six months of age.

not to overfeed your infant. The myth that breastfed infants are protected from obesity later in life is not supported by evidence.

A WORD ABOUT FOOD ALLERGIES

Several years ago, I saw a baby who had been fed peanut butter as one of her initial foods. She came to me with eyelids and face swollen and covered with hives. She survived, but she may be dangerously allergic to any food that contains peanuts for the rest of her life. It remains unclear whether infants "outgrow" their allergy. This is a scientific work in progress. More on peanut butter later.

Other foods associated with allergy in infancy are strawberries, raspberries, fish, shell fish, lobster, shrimp, crab, cinnamon, almonds, walnuts, and eggs - (both egg white and egg yolk should be avoided by infants until over one year). This is one of those revised recommendations. Nutritionists formerly recommended egg yolk because it is rich in iron. What they didn't realize was that iron phosphate, the particular kind of iron found in egg yolk, is absorbed poorly.

For infants with a strong family history of allergies your pediatrician my recommend to further delay the introduction of all the foods mentioned above.

Traditional advice is to introduce a new food and then wait 3 to 7 days before introducing another.[13] The theory is that any allergic reaction will show up during that interval, and the offending food could be identified and eliminated. In all my many years of private practice, I have not found this advice to be of any practical help as long as you avoid the highly allergenic foods, such as peanut butter, nuts, seeds, chocolate, cinnamon,

[13] Nwaru BI et al. Timing of infant feeding in relation to childhood asthma and allergic diseases. *J Allergy Clin Immunol* 2013 Jan; 131:78. (http://dx.doi.org/10.1016/j.jaci.2012.10.028

eggs, berries, lobster, crab, shrimp, and shell fish as I was taught to do by my medical school authorities. Fortunately infants tolerate most other foods extremely well.

Our son married a woman who grew up in Beijing, China. Their daughter is fed the traditional diet of her Chinese mother. My son can't believe what she is fed, and what she loves to eat from food gotten at the Chinese market. At an early age she would try and still enjoys almost any food. This was a positive change from my son, who was and remains a picky eater.

Some studies out of Scandinavia and Israel suggest the opposite, that is, begin introducing these foods early. In the Journal of Clinical Immunology, Jan.2013, the authors report on a Finnish study where investigators followed 3781 Finnish children for 5 years to examine the association between duration of breast-feeding and timing of introduction of complementary foods (based on parent report) and the development of allergic disease and sensitization to foods and inhalants. Introduction of wheat, rye, oats, and barley before age 5.5 months, fish before age 9 months, and egg before age 11 months was associated with lower rates of asthma, allergic rhinitis, and sensitization. Total breast-feeding duration of 9.5 months or more was associated with lower risk for non-atopic asthma, and the benefit seemed to correlate with the duration of total breast-feeding rather than exclusive breast-feeding.

COMMENT: By telling parents for years to delay the introduction of allergenic complementary foods, we might have caused more harm than good. On the basis of these results and recent guidelines (J Allergy Clin Immunol: In Practice 2013;1:29), I recommend exclusive breast-feeding for only 4 months followed by continued breast-feeding with complementary foods until age 12 months. Grains should be started at age 4 months, followed by all other foods during the first year. A recent randomized trial showed similar growth rates and better iron status in breast-fed infants when complementary grains were started at 4 versus 6 months of age. (JW Pediatr Adolesc Med Jan 9 2013)

Dr. Amrol is an Associate Professor of Clinical Internal Medicine and Director of the Division of Allergy and Immunology at the University of South Carolina School of Medicine.
Published in Journal Watch Pediatrics and Adolescent Medicine *January 30, 2013*

There is more evidence at this time, but not enough to make any firm recommendations. Discuss this information with your pediatrician before introducing these foods.

Now having said that, I must say my Vietnamese patients are often fed fish soup beginning at 6-9 months of age. This is a cultural practice, and it is common for different cultures to follow their traditional approach to infant feeding. For example, the Indian infant who is often fed by the grandmother, gives her grandchild what was given to her as an infant. With success!

Another food to be avoided until the baby is over one year, (although not an allergen) is honey, as it has been linked to infant botulism. Botulism causes muscle weakness in infancy, often beginning with facial weakness, droopy eyelids, or the loss of ability to sit. Constipation is another early sign of infant botulism. If not treated early it can cause paralysis of the muscles needed for breathing. Although this is a rare condition, should you ever suspect it in your infant, call your physician immediately and tell him or her of your concern.

WHEAT, MILK AND OTHER FOOD INTOLERANCES

In the 1960's, when an infant had persistent diarrhea, a popular diagnosis was celiac disease or gluten - induced intolerance. The baby was immediately taken off any wheat products (and foods containing **gliadin** - the protein found in wheat, rye, oats, barley, and buckwheat which is responsible for this illness). In fact, celiac disease was until recently thought to be a rare illness. We know that certain viruses can cause prolonged diarrhea, and the parasitic infection, **giardiasis** mimics many of the symptoms of celiac disease, with foul smelling bowel movements, gas, and abdominal pain. Most of those infants in the 60's may have been wheat or gluten intolerant or were temporarily intolerant to wheat, milk and juice as a result of an intestinal infection. The key word is **temporary.** Today we have a simple blood test to determine whether a child's belly pains are due to celiac disease. My granddaughter was diagnosed with "acid reflux" as a cause of her persistent bellyaches or, "Stress." Finally she was tested for celiac disease and her test was extremely positive. This was confirmed by biopsy at the university hospital. Since the diagnosis and dietary changes, she has grown many inches, is now smiling, and as long as she follows a gluten free diet, she has very few bellyaches.

Milk sugar (lactose) intolerance in infancy is highly unusual except briefly after a viral diarrhea. Nevertheless many babies are unnecessarily taken off milk formula and put on an elemental formula for their entire first year. It appears that parents, grandparents, and some physicians blame milk or teething for any unexplained crankiness or fever in infancy.

ABOUT FRUIT AND VEGETABLES

Another common recommendation is to start fruit before vegetables. There is little scientific information to support what order is best. Pediatricians do almost as well as grandmothers when it comes to choosing first foods. Almost all schedules are speculative, intuitive or anecdotal. The message is, You decide!

Apples and pears are popular fruits, and most babies tolerate them quite well. Cooked carrots, squash, yams, and potato are foods I personally recommend to my patients. If these are tolerated I suggest adding peas, strained spinach, beets, beans, broccoli, and Brussels sprouts. However, I'm not dogmatic about the order in which foods are introduced. The choice is yours. That's part of the fun of being a parent.

I have more concern about the practice of adding a little salt[14] or sugar to the baby's food, whether done by the commercial baby food company or the parent. In Europe, Asia, Central and South America, parents introduce soups at an early age. They put all these vegetables in a broth and mash or blend it into a soup. Infants usually love this and as the baby matures, the soup takes on a more lumpy, stew-like texture. This is a major problem because these soups too often contain added salt plus the amount in the broth. To avoid this, use a non-salted broth[15]and forget the pinch of salt that makes it tasty to your palate! Experiment with textures. Babies without teeth may gum lumpy food easily, while some infants with teeth may gag on the same foods. As the baby matures, more and more textures will be tolerated until eating "grown-up" food cut in small pieces will be eaten exclusively.

When foods aren't pureed, you may notice partially digested material in the bowel movement. This is especially true for corn or raisins and is quite normal. Stool color also changes with different foods. Don't be alarmed if the bowel movement is green. The only colors of concern in B.M.'s are red, jet black, or cream-clay. Red and black may suggest bowel bleeding, while the clay color may be associated with a liver problem. However, colors often reflect the color of the foods eaten such as beets, peas, or spinach. Spinach, by the way, is an excellent natural laxative for infants as well as adults - it's not, however, the fabulous source of iron it's reputed to be. The baby doesn't absorb the iron in spinach as well as in many other iron-rich foods.

---

14 Hypertension 1997;29:913-917,930-936 Dietary Nutrients Early In Life Influence Later Blood Pressure

15 Trader Joe's Organic low sodium Chicken Broth

PROTEIN AND YOUR INFANT

Today, health conscious parents who know that meat, fish or chicken are good sources of protein, wonder if they shouldn't be providing those foods to their baby. They often think of milk as a "calcium" food and forget that it is also very rich in protein. In fact, a 13 - pound infant requires only 12-13 grams of protein daily, which is easily provided by breastfeeding or feeding three eight-ounce bottles of formula a day. The reason for suggesting the introduction of the above foods is not necessarily because of their protein content, but because they are an excellent source of the much needed mineral iron. There is little clinical evidence against beginning meats as a first food. It's your baby, so you decide what your first foods will be!

The fatty acids, ARA and DHA (see "Nutrition 101" for more in depth details) are also found in fish and are important in eye and brain development. My mother used to tell me that fish was a "brain food" and encouraged me to eat it as a young child. Now it appears that she may have been correct.

But remember, fish is a potent allergen, so consult with your healthcare provider before introducing it.

After one year of age, when the baby switches to cow milk, more protein will be provided than mother's milk or formula. In fact, three 8 oz. cups or bottles of cow milk a day contain enough protein for infants up to 30 pounds. So there's really no need to worry about insufficient protein. Because cow milk is iron-poor, it's important to introduce iron-rich foods, as explained earlier, and to make vegetables a significant part of the daily diet. I don't recommend ham, bacon, sausage, hot dogs, or lunch meats because of their high salt, saturated fat and nitrite content. There are better choices to obtain important nutrients than from these "holiday foods." Partially cooked meats are dangerous because thorough cooking is needed to kill contaminating bacteria or parasites that can cause deadly diarrhea by E. coli, salmonella-shigella, and campylobacter, as well as the diseases toxoplasmosis, trichinosis or tapeworms.

Some nutritionists recommend beef or chicken liver as a good source of iron and vitamins. It is true that liver contains many important nutrients, but I no longer recommend liver as a nutritional source. As a detoxifying organ the liver may contain a high concentration of all sorts of environmental poisons. There are safer ways to obtain these nutrients. I don't feel good about feeding liver to infants or children, and that includes the popular liverwurst sandwich.

OTHER CAUTIONARY NOTES

Plain pasteurized yogurt, Greek yogurt and cottage cheese are fine foods, (unless filled with added sugar as in Yoplait[16] and some "fruit" Greek or non-fat yogurts) but since your less than one-year old infant is already consuming a lot of milk, he or she doesn't need either from a nutritional standpoint. Concentrating on vegetables is preferable and healthier.

The emphasis on dairy foods is a product of the National Dairy Council's biased promotion of dairy to nutrition programs at schools and the university level. In fact, there is some suggestion and concern that dairy is over-consumed in the Western Diet.

Do not give your baby raw carrots, popcorn, peanuts, grapes, or other similarly hard to chew foods. I don't recommend popcorn or peanuts until the child is four years old or older. An infant can choke to death on a grape, or inhale a tiny bit of food into the lungs and end up with pneumonia. The hot dog remains the most common cause of choking death.

I've heard of letting a baby teethe on a cold carrot, but the carrot won't dissolve in the throat if the infant is choking on it.

[16] Yoplait-6 oz contains a total of 7 teaspoon of sugar, of which 3 teaspoons are from added sugar.

A piece of zwieback or unsalted rice cake is preferable for teething foods. Teething rings are of little value and sales are aimed mostly to keep anxious parents occupied.

Some parents let infants eat crackers as finger foods. This is okay as long as you check the contents for salt, saturated fat and sugar. Graham crackers are high in sugar or honey. It sticks to the older child's teeth and contributes to early caries.

Now is the time to make your house safe. Not only do you need safety locks but you need to convert your house into a **Nutritionally Safe Home**. Control what foods are in the home. Yes, I know, your husband wants all that junk food and ice cream in the freezer! And, yes, you have another child who is skinny. This is the first step toward preventing your child from the addiction to fat, salt and sugar. If you are serious about providing optimal nutrition to you child, then it is time to consider changing your home into a less toxic environment. Before you know it, your child will be entering school and this advice will no longer be practical. It is much easier to prevent habits than to break them.

In a safe house, limit or avoid totally: pickles, canned fruit, macaroni and cheese, Goldfish, doughnuts, "fresh squeezed organic juices" (they contain more sugar than Coke), and sugary cereals masquerading as food. Remember, if it has a Nutrition Facts label, it most likely is processed. Buy real foods, vegetables, fruit, and don't forget fish, lean meats, poultry, milk and eggs.

Many commercial crackers contain 40% of their calories from fat and are loaded with salt. Although I'm not worried about the fat content during infancy, this is when habits begin. It has been demonstrated that a low salt diet in infancy protects against the development of high blood pressure later in life.[17] High blood

[17] Hypertension 1997; Dietary Nutrients Early In Life Influence Later Blood Pressure. This study warns us that a high sodium diet "in utero (during pregnancy) and in infancy may be more important in relation to cardiovascular disease than exposures in adulthood, as 'programming' of different systems and organs in the body occurs very early in life."

pressure later in life may well be the price we pay for too much salt in childhood.

FOOD NOTES ON LIQUIDS OTHER THAN MILK

It's nutritionally more sound to give the baby water than juice.[18] If you choose to give juice, be certain that it is pasteurized, if not fresh, and limit it to only once a week. If your baby totes a bottle around all day for security, do not put diluted juice in it. Use pure water. Tap water is fine. If your water is not fluoridated and you don't use a fluoride supplement, bottled fluoridated water is a good option. It is healthier and won't destroy the infant's teeth or appetite for healthier foods.

I've seen many two-year-olds whose teeth were nearly rotted away from the ever-present bottle of diluted apple juice. And premature loss of primary teeth lead can lead to damage in the permanent teeth. Because milk sugar, lactose, promotes cavities, rotting teeth is seen in breastfeeding babies over a year of age when the mother uses her breasts as a pacifier.

Orange and other citrus juices can cause a contact rash around the mouth. The fresher the juice, the more **peel oil** is present in the juice. It is the peel oils that cause the irritation to the skin around the mouth, not citric acid. This is not allergy. Tomato sauce also contains a lot of peel oil, and also may cause skin irritation. If you wash the infant's face immediately after feeding foods with high peel oil content, these rashes may be

[18] Although 70% of parents with infants 6 months and under say they give juice to their babies, there is no nutritional need for it. Fruit juice lacks the protein, fat, calories, calcium, vitamin D, iron and zinc needed to support normal development in infancy and childhood. The vitamin C in fruit itself is a more nutritious source than juice, and mother's milk has plenty of vitamin C as well. Infant formulas are fortified with vitamin C. How often have you seen Scurvy? Many juices have as much as 6 teaspoons of sugar (24 grams) in a small container.

avoided or decreased. Peel oil concentrations are controlled in the commercial production of all juices. Today formulas are fortified with Vitamin C, and many non-citrus juices are too. Breast milk contains sufficient Vitamin C to protect your infant from scurvy.

Multivitamin drops that contain vitamin A,D, and C plus iron are recommended for most infants.

In the early 1970's, I had an epidemic of yellow-orange babies in my practice. It wasn't jaundice - the whites of their eyes were clear, and the babies were vigorous - it was too much beta-carotene from carrot juice. Once they drank less carrot juice, the color disappeared. Carotene is also found in squash, sweet potato, and tomato. The color does not harm the baby. The real problem with carrot juice is that an important nutrient, fiber, is discarded during processing. Health conscious parents often try to avoid processed foods, and inadvertently do the processing themselves. There are now juicers available that retain the fiber and those are the preferred types. Fiber slows the absorption of the carrot sugars, but some nutritionist claim that blenders defeat the delaying effect of fiber. That is why I recommend smoothies to be served only once a week at most.

Prune juice is well tolerated by most infants and toddlers and is high in iron, but I haven't found it to be especially effective for constipation. Prunes or plums seem to have better results as natural laxatives for infants and children. If you prepare your own, look for prunes (at most health food stores) that don't contain sulfites[19] as a preservative. If your child needs a natural laxative, figs, brown rice, spinach, and peas are excellent additional helpers.

Cola drinks, regular and diet soda, Kool Aid, Hi - C, Gatorade, sports and energy drinks, or punch have no place in an infant's diet. Or for that matter, in older children or teens. Carbonated beverages do not "settle" an upset stomach, and Gatorade is not good for an infant with diarrhea or dehydration. Sodas contain

[19] Sulfites can cause minor and sometimes severe allergic reactions.

lots sugar and in addition, phosphate, a compound that promotes calcium loss. This is hardly a time in an infant's development when that should happen.

Don't feed non-pasteurized eggnog or raw egg, honey and banana blended as a milk shake - an "old wives'" solution for putting weight on infants. Raw eggs often contain the salmonella germ and may also be very allergenic. Raw egg poses far more danger to the infant than low weight.

It's fine to give traditional breakfast foods for dinner and the vegetables, meat, and potatoes for breakfast. Most arrangements are cultural. Many Asian babies eat fish and rice for breakfast. The main meal in South and Central America is lunch. Furthermore, foods can be given more than once a day. In fact, many infants go on jags-preferring a particular food for days or weeks, then suddenly reject the food entirely and demand something they wouldn't touch the week before. Don't let such temperamental tastes discourage you from reintroducing a rejected food on another day.

Commercially prepared baby foods are now being promoted as first step and second step foods. This is a marketing tactic. The latter is often referred to as junior foods. The difference between these foods is texture, not nutritional value. In fact, sugar is often added to these baby foods, so check the ingredients before purchasing them. They are designed to help the infant achieve a smooth transition to table foods. Generally second step foods are started at about 7 to 8 months of age; however, the age at which infants accept the more coarse texture is highly variable. Some children resist these lumpy foods until the end of the first year or even later. Do not feel that you must switch from strained foods.

You and your infant will decide how much of each food is appropriate. Don't force a baby to finish the jar or an arbitrary portion you've prepared. As a new father, I remember the games I made up to get that last teaspoon of food into my daughter's mouth. "Here comes the airplane into the hanger!" And just as I was congratulating myself on my slick maneuver, she'd gag and throw up the entire meal!

SALT: IS IT TRULY THE WHITE DEATH?

Salt or sodium chloride, is one of our oldest food preservatives, used in commercially prepared foods as an inexpensive way to inhibit molds, retard spoilage, and provide smooth texture and quick-cooking properties. It's also a necessary mineral in our diet. On food labels, the words **sodium, soda,** monosodium glutamate, or the chemical symbol for sodium, **Na.**, all signify **salt.** An infant's preference for salt does not emerge until four months, but how much is innate and how much is learned remains uncertain - quite unlike our taste for sugar, with which we seem to be born.

Too much salt in childhood is an extreme dietary hazard, and has been linked to the development of hypertension (high blood pressure) in teenagers and adults.[20] A high salt diet beginning in infancy is a major cause of high blood pressure in adulthood. In a Dutch study, newborns who were fed, in addition to breast milk, formula and foods providing 22mg of sodium a day had lower blood pressures than those fed diets with 58 mg a day. Fifteen years after the study ended, the difference in blood pressure was still there.[21]

[20] Journal of Hypertension 14 (suppl.): S210, 1996

[21] In the past few years there have been a few studies, mostly subsidized by the food industry, claiming that the effect of sodium as a cause of high blood pressure has been greatly exaggerated. The researchers are from reputable universities, but these seriously flawed studies have been very short term. Totally ignored in these studies are infants, children and young adults. Newspapers, magazines and "health journals" have been publishing outrageous distortions under headlines suggesting salt should be used more liberally and that our prior understanding of salt or sodium is now obsolete dogma. No wonder most people are confused when presented with such disinformation. Chefs from major restaurants are already featuring dishes enhanced with flavors from exotic "healthy"salts.

While high blood pressure seems to run in some families, lots of sodium helps encourage this undesirable family trait. Whether or not there is any history of high blood pressure[22] or stroke in your family, I recommend you limit your child's sodium intake - and your own.

The amount of sodium in a diet should approximate a ratio of sodium in milligrams (mg.) to the amount of calories in your diet. Therefore, a 700-calorie diet should have sodium limited to about 700mg of sodium, while a 2000-calorie diet should limit sodium intake to 2000mg or two grams.[23] Avoid foods with more than 350 mg of sodium per serving. The right amount of sodium needed by children through adulthood can be found **naturally** in fresh vegetables, grains, meats, poultry, and fish. But in fact, many children consume over 5000 mg of sodium daily while adults often consume from 10,000 to 12,000 milligrams **daily** between what's natural in the food, what the food industry has added to the food, and what we add ourselves from the salt shaker in the kitchen and at the table!

When selecting a food, note the amount of calories. Then check the label for sodium content[24]. If the sodium content in

[22] High blood pressure is a serious matter. What a child eats sets the stage for high blood pressure later in life. It can eventually lead to heart failure, a condition where the heart gets larger and weaker and is less able to pump blood. High blood pressure can also lead to aneurysms. Aneurysms are small blister-like areas in the blood vessels of the brain (leading to a stroke) or the aorta which can burst, (dissecting aortic artery) causing rapid death or permanent disability. Kidney failure is another result of high blood pressure. As blood vessels in the kidney narrow, they are less able to supply the kidney with blood.. This could lead to permanent kidney damage. High blood pressure also speeds the hardening of arteries. Healthy arteries are elastic. When the arteries to the brain, heart and other organs become less elastic or hard, they are less able to carry blood and the result is early aging or premature death of these organs.

[23] One teaspoon of table salt equals 6375 milligrams of table salt. 6375 mg of table salt = 2400 mg sodium. One teaspoon of table salt contains 2400 milligrams sodium.

[24] A cup of cottage cheese, a small bag of pretzels, and a salad with Italian

milligrams is far above the number of calories, search the shelves for a brand that contains less salt. There are many canned soups available now that have a reduced or low salt counterpart. Bread and cheese are very high salt foods. Check the labels - you'll be surprised. Take time out one day to calculate how much salt you actually consume in a day. The figure may be shocking!

For most Americans, 10% of the sodium in their diet occurs naturally in food, 15% comes from the salt they shake on while cooking or at the table, and 75% is added to food during processing. A bowl of canned chicken noodle soup can deliver 900 mg of sodium–for a child, that's over a day's worth of sodium and that's why it's so important to check the Nutrition Facts label.

Children in a nationally representative sample consumed an average of 3,387 mgs of sodium per day, more than double the upper limit of 1500 mgs recommended.

The Recommended Dietary Allowance (RDA) of sodium for healthy adults is 2,300 mg daily. That is equivalent to one teaspoon (6375mg) of salt a day. The children's RDA for sodium are the following:

Ages 2-3 is 1000 mgs
Ages 4-8 is 1200 mgs
Ages 9-18 is 1500 mgs

If you can save your child from the habit of craving a relatively high salt diet, you may save him or her from future heart disease or stroke, or an earlier death. I personally know many middle aged men and women who ignored this advice and have suffered a possibly preventable brain damaging stroke.[25]

---

dressing is more than the adult recommended daily limit of sodium–2400mg! A glass of tomato juice contains 880mg and the parmesan cheese sprinkled on top of a pasta dinner adds about 500mg

25 A stroke is a "brain attack" and its mechanism is similar to a "heart attack." Blood vessels to the brain either burst or become blocked. The stroke is referred to as a hemorrhagic stroke if it is caused by a burst blood vessel to the brain, or an ischemic stroke if it is due to a blocked blood vessel. Ischemic stroke is the most common. In both cases, damage to the brain is caused by

Improve your odds by modifying your own salt intake. The following is a five-step program for the gradual reduction of salt in your family's diet. It takes most adults about a year to withdraw from the salt craving. Go slowly and you won't feel deprived. It will take the children much less time, but in either case it's a minor and brief deprivation in the big scheme of things, and worth it.

FIVE STEPS FOR MODIFYING SALT INTAKE

1. Empty the salt from the shaker on the table, and refill with a non-sodium herbal substitute.

2. Gradually use less salt in cooking - don't use it at all in cooking water. Start with half the salt a recipe calls for. After a few months, omit salt for cooking entirely.

3. Notice sodium content on food labels. Canned foods are very high in sodium (unless specifically stated as, "reduced sodium, low sodium or no salt added"), followed by frozen foods; but some fresh foods are too – such as tomato and celery- therefore don't add salt to such dishes. REFER TO THE SECTION ON "READING FOOD LABELS."

---

lack of oxygen and blood glucose. Oxygen and glucose are essential nutrients carried to the brain by blood vessels. Brain cells quickly begin to die without these nutrients. The results may be impaired speech if the brain cells in the speech center die; paralysis of the arms or legs if the motor brain cells die; blindness if the vision center brain cells die or coma and death if the stroke is severe enough to cause the death of enough vital brain cells. A diet low in sodium and saturated fat plus regular exercise greatly reduces the risk of stroke. Although stroke is usually an event that occurs in adulthood, its roots (poor eating and exercise habits) are developed during childhood.

4. Don't keep highly salted foods in the house. Avoid the temptation of buying high sodium crackers, chips, salted nuts, bacon, sausages, lunch meats, dehydrated soups, tomato or V-8 juice, most canned soups, pickles, relishes, barbecue sauces, lox, herring, many processed cheeses and especially cheddar cheeses, or Jell-O. Treat yourself to such foods only on special occasions in small amounts, when you're away from home or at a Super Bowl party.

5. In a year's time you won't believe how different foods taste, or that you ever purposefully put salt on your corn on the cob! Restaurant food may seem very salty, unless you ask the chef to use very little salt and no MSG.

WHAT ABOUT SUGAR?

When we think of sugar, we generally imagine that white crystalline product - but that's just the tip of the sugar iceberg. Sugar exists in most foods we eat: juice, soda, jams, cookies, chocolate, crackers, hot and dry cereals, pies, ice cream, chili, pizza, Jell-O, hot dogs, bacon, ham, salami, and cold cuts, stuffings, breads, soups, mayonnaise, catsup, salad dressing, fruit flavored yogurt, canned vegetables, beans, and virtually all frozen foods, to name just a few. The average American consumed approximately 120 lbs. of sugar a year in 1998 which is a tremendous amount. It must be 50% more now in 2013!

Besides refined cane and beet sugar, chemically know as sucrose, check food labels for refined fructose, glucose, dextrose, lactose, levulose, maltose. All of these refined sugars have been stripped of their mineral, vitamin, and fiber content. They are good as a sweetener and for calories; whereas nutritious foods such as oranges, blackberries, blueberries, strawberries, cantaloupe, apples, plums, papaya, mango, and dried fruits are all high in sugar but retain the important vitamins, minerals, and fiber. The sugar in these foods is absorbed more slowly by the body than with refined sugars or juices. Other refined sugars such as corn syrup, molasses, maple syrup, and honey are absorbed rapidly and stress the hormones in our body that maintain balance or homeostasis. "Sugarless" desserts and ice cream are sometimes deceptively loaded with honey or "real maple syrup." Although many parents or children may prefer a particular type of sugar, the body uses all sugars in essentially the same way. None of these sugars are nutritionally better than cane sugars, and brown sugar, raw sugar, honey, or molasses are not any healthier than other sugars.

Apple juice is probably the greatest source of sugar in a small child's diet. It should be limited to a single 6 oz. bottle or cup a week, (**at the most**) but not toted around in the bottle. "Watered-down" juice is very popular, but is especially damaging to the teeth and appetite when consumed throughout the day (and night). Baby food companies cunningly promote juice by **strategically placing rows of juice bottles above the desirable baby fruit and vegetable jars!** **An infant has no nutritional need for juice.** Formula and breast milk provide an infant with enough water even in hot weather. Breast milk also contains lots of sugar (lactose or milk sugar). Infants that breastfeed past a year of age, especially as a calming agent, all day and throughout the night, often develop severely decayed teeth. This habit can lead to diseased permanent teeth.

The impact on behavior from eating sugar and various foods has been a topic of both interest and concern to parents. There is now considerable evidence that the concern about sugar consumption as reflected by the media was in error. The myths surrounding sugar, including the myth of the "sugar high" or that it causes hyperactivity, has been slow to disappear. These myths are misleading and harmful. We need to place sugar in the diet in perspective. Small amounts of sugar have an important place in nutrition. For example, the only fuel the brain uses is sugar. Actually there is some evidence showing sugar to have a calming[26] effect on normal and hyperactive children. Too much sugar, on the other hand, such as too much of anything, is detrimental to our health and eating too much sugar does contribute to tooth decay, obesity, constipation, malnutrition, and the metabolic syndrome .[27] A major issue is that there is no RDA for sugar. So when one says, "A little bit" what does that mean?

The average American consumes 45 gallons of sugary drinks a year. A 20oz. bottle of soda contains 16 teaspoons of sugar and this is a huge contributor to obesity, heart disease, diabetes, and tooth decay. Now that is not, "a little bit."

Fructose and high fructose corn syrup (HFCS) are in the headlines now and for good reason. Fructose may be the driver of metabolic syndrome. Sucrose breaks down into glucose and our enemy fructose. Are these sugars toxic? Are they addictive? The evidence is mounting and sugar is ubiquitous. Even Gerber and Heinz add sugars to more than half of their Second Stage and Third State fruit and some vegetables. Sport juices and fruit juices, berry juices along with sodas line the supermarkets and grocery stores. Are these poisons? I don't know, but my recom-

---

[26] Facts and myths about sugar. Department of Nutritional Sciences Faculty of Medicine, University of Toronto, Ontario, Canada. Bol Asoc Med P R 1991 Sep;83(9); 408-10. Effects of diets high in sucrose or aspartame on the behavior and cognitive performance of children. Department of Pediatrics, Vanderbilt University, Nashville, TN , N Engl J Med 1994 Feb 3; 330(5):301-7.

Effect of sugar on aggresive and inattentive behavior in children with attention deficit disorder with hyperactivty and normal children. Wender EH, Solanto MV: Schneider Children's Hospital, Long Island Jewish Medical Center, New Hyde Park, New York 11042. Pediatrics 1991 Nov:88(5): 960-6.

[27] The metabolic syndrome is the name for a group of risk factors, such as obesity, that raise your risk for heart disease and diabetes. This will be discussed in greater detail later in this book.

Effect of nutritional supplements on attention-deficit hyperactivity disorder. Dykman KD, Dykman RA. Integr Physiol Behav. Sci 1998 Jan-Mar;33(1)49-60.

mendation is to keep these drinks out of your home and out of your food except for special holidays and occasions.

We are now in the midst of an obesity epidemic. Much of it is a result of consuming high sugar drinks, overeating and lack of exercise. Many of my obese and overweight patients confess to drinking 6-8 large sodas, sugar drinks or juice a day. That's well over 50 teaspoons of sugar a day and that does not include the sugar from their ice cream, candy bars, energy bars and multiple other sources. When I go to the

movies I see the long lines leading up to the "food" concession where super sized drinks, ice cream, hot dogs, pizza, chips, nachos, and giant sized candy bars are sold. Once in the theater the screen reminds us there is still time to get some more. Don't starve or become dehydrated during a tense 2 hour movie!

As they say, "A second in your mouth, a minute in the stomach, and the rest of your life (as fat) on your hips, butt, and gut!" Think of that before taking your first bite. Let's face it, who can eat only one or two potato chips and then put the bag away. Better to resist the first bite. If you are not able to follow this advice, seek out a 12 step program.

MAKING YOUR OWN BABY FOODS

▲ ▲ ▲

If you have the time, making your baby food at home is a way to really be in charge of your infant's nutrition and may save money.

DO: Home preparation of baby foods requires special attention to cleanliness. Be sure to wash your hands with soap and water before handling food. Always use a clean cutting board and knife. Thoroughly wash, peel, and trim all fruit and vegetables to remove soil and unwanted food contaminants such as pesticides and chemical residues.[28] Although some authorities recommend using detergents to wash fruit and vegetables, I don't, because I'm concerned about adding residues to the foods from these detergents. Avoid using ceramic or glazed containers unless you are certain that they do not contain lead. Lead poisoning may

[28] The 1995 annual report of California's Department of Pesticide Regulations reports that more than 98% of the produce sampled by the state had "either no detectable residues or residues within legal limits." The benefits of eating ample amounts of fruits and vegetables far outweigh health risks posed by the low amounts of pesticide residues.

result if lead is leached out from these bowls and contaminate the food.

Ceramic salad bowl from Mexico or Central America often contain traces of lead. The vinegar in salad may leach out traces of lead. Better to avoid such bowls for use and keep them as ornaments.

DON'T: Don't add salt or seasonings or use salted leftovers. Don't add sugar or honey. (Don't add any seasonings to commercially prepared food either!) It doesn't have to taste good to you; just to baby!

TOOLS YOU'LL NEED

Since you'll be pureeing most of the baby's food to a consistency he or she can swallow, you'll need a manual food mill or electric baby food grinder (available in most department stores), or a blender, or food processor, or a strainer with a wooden spoon. Babies' preferences for textures vary from fine to lumpy - this is true before and after their teeth come in. Your infant will let you know what consistency is preferred - don't feel you have to rush through purees to chunky foods.

STORING HOMEMADE FOODS

Refrigerate uneaten food promptly. Discard pureed foods after 15 - 24 hours of refrigeration. It's safe to freeze most baby food for one to two months; but once a container is thawed or partially used, leftovers should be discarded. These rules also apply to commercially prepared baby foods.

Some people store pureed foods in Zip-Loc or baby bottle type bags and freeze them; others pour the puree into BPA free[29] ice cube trays, freeze it, and then slip the cubes into freezer bags to store. Later several frozen cubes can be heated in a pan or microwave oven. Label all bags including the date of preparation.

USE OF MICROWAVE OVENS

It is unsafe to microwave infant formula because the fluid continues to cook even after it is removed from the oven and can burn the baby's mouth. Most other baby foods can be warmed safely in a microwave oven by heating for only a few seconds. Baby foods should be **warmed** to room temperature and not made **hot**. Microwave heating is very uneven. The container may feel cool, but it may contain pockets of food at scalding temperature. Stir the food thoroughly after heating to even out the temperature and be sure to recheck the temperature before offering it to your baby.

PREPARING FRUIT

Infants are born with a "sweet tooth" even before their teeth come in (mother's milk contains a large amount of natural sugar), so most fruits are well received. But beware of allergic reactions - strawberries and other berries should be avoided during infancy.

[29] Bisphenol A (BPA) is a controversial chemical that can be found in the lining of some food cans, certain plastic water bottles, infant feeding plastic bottles and more. Some researchers have linked this hormone-mimicking chemical to a host of issues including behavioral and developmental effect in children. Only use BPA free containers.

Avoid polycarbonate cups or bottles and do not heat beverages or food in any kind of plastic container. Some advertised microwave-safe containers my leach out BPA into food from packaging.

And be aware of possible side effects: some fruits, such as orange or tomato, which have high concentrations of peel oil, can cause a rash to sensitive skin. Wipe the baby's lips and chin with warm water and a soft cloth after feeding such foods.

BANANA PUREE

Wrap a peeled banana in foil.

- Bake at 400 degrees F for 15-20 minutes or microwave a banana (without foil) until it achieves a very soft mushy consistency. Experiment with the time it takes in your particular microwave. The microwave oven is safe to use in the preparation of foods. In fact, microwaving fruit and vegetables destroys fewer vitamins and other nutrients than boiling, steaming or baking. In all the recipes that follow, the instructions may be modified for microwave preparation.

- Mash or blend to desired consistency. Add a little formula or breast milk to improve texture and make it thinner if needed.

APPLES, PEACHES, APRICOTS, PEARS, AND PLUMS

- Wash fruit well.

- Peel[30] (except for plums and apricots), remove seeds, pit and slice fruit.

[30] If you peel and discard fruit skins such as apple or pear, remember that there is a trade-off: you may reduce pesticide residue somewhat, but lose dietary fiber

- Put fruit in boiling water. (Use 1 TBS of water per cup of peaches or plums, 2 TBS of water per cup of apples, apricots, and pears.)

- Simmer apples, pears, and peaches for 15-20 minutes. Cook plums and apricots for 35-40 minutes. Remove plum skins.

- When fruit is soft, blend for about 30 seconds, or mash until smooth.

You can store these fruits in the freezer for up to two months.

PREPARING VEGGIES

Most babies enjoy carrots, squash, broccoli, cauliflower, peas, and yams, and all these make nutritious first foods. Buy certified organic foods when they are available. This will decrease the probability of pesticides or chemical residues.

The general rules for cooking vegetables for adults also applies to infants: Wash all vegetables thoroughly to remove soil and any trace of pesticide. Don't use too much water when you steam the vegetables - about one third of a cup of water per pound of vegetables is enough.

Add vegetables after the water is boiling, then cover and cook over medium-low heat until vegetables are tender. Don't overcook so that vegetables are mushy. Set aside the cooking water, now rich in vitamins, to mix with your mashed or blended or pureed vegetables to thin to the desired consistency.

Pour into BPA free ice cube tray and freeze. Then slip out cubes and store them in a freezer bag.

CARROTS

- Peel, slice, and boil in a covered pot for 10-20 minutes. Grind or blend to desired consistency.

SQUASH

- Slice and boil SUMMER SQUASH for 5-15 minutes, WINTER SQUASH for 15-20 minutes in a covered pot. Puree.

BROCCOLI AND CAULIFLOWER

- Boil 15-20 minutes in a covered pot. Puree to desired consistency.

PEAS

- Boil for 10-15 minutes in a covered pot. Puree.

YAMS, SWEET POTATOES, REGULAR POTATOES

- Peel and quarter.
- Boil in a covered pot (add a little more water than for the vegetables above) for 15-20 minutes, then puree.
- In the case of yams and potatoes, discard the cooking water and add formula, or breast milk to thin your puree.

BEANS

Garbonzo beans, baby lima beans, navy, pinto, red kidney beans, and lentils are all popular with babies, but some parents postpone their introduction until the infant is 12-15 months old because of beans' association with gassiness. But most of my Latin American patients offer them earlier with no problems. One cup of dry beans make two and one half cups of cooked beans.

- Wash beans well.

- Boil one cup of dried beans in 4 cups of water for two or three hours, depending on the variety of bean.[31]

- Blend or puree using the cooking water to thin,

- Or the beans may be mashed in a non-stick pan with chopped onion and cilantro, then "refried."

STRAINED MEATS AND POULTRY

(Begin these foods after the baby has learned to enjoy a variety of vegetables)

A blender isn't really sufficient for preparing meat and poultry for your baby. You'll need a food processor, electric baby food grinder, or manual grinder.

Strained meats and poultry may be kept frozen for about two months.

---

[31] Most of my Latin American (especially Central American and Mexican) parents do not soak beans overnight. The practice decreases cooking time, but a busy parent may omit this step. Other parents find it easier to soak the beans overnight rather than watching them an additional two hours to prevent scorching.

CHICKEN OR TURKEY

- Boil or bake chicken or turkey as usual.
- Remove cooked chicken or turkey from bones; discard skin.
- Grind or blend meat in processor, adding some of the liquid in which you boiled or baked the meat to achieve the consistency your baby likes.

BEEF OR VEAL

- Use only lean beef or veal, and remove all visible fat.
- Boil veal for about 40 minutes, beef for 2 1/2 hours.
- Grind or blend cooked meat in food processor, using cooking liquid for combining to the right consistency.

GENERAL PRINCIPLES IN THE CREATION OF SOUPS

Although most of my parents do not introduce soups until their children are two years old or older, Latin and Asian children are often given soup before age one.

- Start with a no-salt added broth. (canned or home made.)
- There are hundreds of broth recipes available, so I have not included one here.)
- To boiling broth add any or all of the following :

Peas, carrots, potato, broccoli, choyote,[32] chopped tomato, small pieces of chicken, cut up pieces of meat and onion, cilantro or parsley if desired. **Do not be afraid to be creative.**

Mash or blend the added vegetables and meats and return them to the soup. Younger children enjoy the nutritious broth and as they get older, begin eating the more textured ingredients. **Do not add salt!**

[32] Chayote, also called mirliton or choko, is a gourd-like squash that is about the size and shape of a very large pear. The skin is pale green and smooth with slight ridges that run lengthwise. Many compare the color to a light green apple. The flesh is white and there is one soft seed in the middle. Chayote is grown in the US in several states including California, Florida, and Louisiana, and throughout South and East Asia, where they are harvested much larger than in the Americas, but it is native to Latin America. Historically, this squash was one of the primary foods of the Aztecs and Mayas.

FEEDING YOUR TODDLER OR PRESCHOOLER

▲ ▲ ▲

WHAT IS FAST FOOD?

Fast food is a food high in calories, sugar, fat, salt, and often caffeine. It is highly processed, "energy dense" and designed to be highly tasty. Many of the nutrients and fiber have been removed during processing. Lots of sugar and salt is added to improve flavor. In addition these foods are conveniently packaged and highly advertised to children and parents over TV hundred of times a day appealing to busy parents to buy these foods for their children's lunch box. Pre-schools and hospitals unwittingly promote these foods from their vending machines. If you wish to see how FAST FOODS have invaded our healthcare system, go to any hospital children's ward and take a look in their refrigerator! Thus a pattern is set early in life and often leads to addiction to junk food. Food preferences are formed before kids ever go to school. They get hooked on sugar at an early age

and it becomes difficult to kick the habit with age. Prevention is easier than treatment of (fast food) junk food addiction.

As witness to this is the epidemic of childhood and adult obesity. Marin County is not insulated from this epidemic. Especially hit are the poor and recent immigrants. It is reported that American-born children of immigrants tend to have shorter lifespans than their parents. American-style behaviors, such as eating high calorie diets and not getting enough exercise may be the blame. According to one study, Latin-American immigrants live almost 3 years longer than American-born Hispanics!

TODDLERS' TABLE FOODS

Most children begin to eat table foods at between one and two years, which gives you one or two years from the baby's birth to clean up your nutritional act. Because even though you think you won't feed your toddler the kind of junk food you indulge in, she's almost certain to have other ideas. Babies especially desire the foods they see their parent eating. In no time at all, your valiant efforts - the careful nursing, home made baby foods, conscientious avoidance of salt and extra sugars, reading all those labels - can come to nothing when your baby gets into your bag of potato chips or Gold Fish.

Not only must you watch what you eat, you must watch what you don't eat. If you turn up your nose at broccoli or fish, your child is likely to do the same. Interestingly, for some reason children seem to emulate their fathers' food habits in particular. So fathers beware: you're the role model!

Babies at the toddler stage love finger foods. Get ready for spilled food, cereal mushed in the baby's hair and slathered all over his face, clothes and your furniture. It's one big sticky mess for the next year or two!

Save the carpet by putting a plastic sheet under the high chair, or enlist a pet dog. But save your energy trying to teach table manners until the baby has developed better fine-motor coordination at about two-and-a-half to three years of age. When eating dissolves into playing, consider ending the meal promptly and allowing the child to leave the table. Some toddlers are not yet ready for exclusive self-feeding. These children need help if they do not eat enough alone. There are children at this age who won't eat at all unless they are fed. Don't become upset, children vary in their readiness. In addition, some children are slow or pokey eaters. When they are rushed, they may leave the table before they're full, and go away hungry. I see this behavior often in kindergarten children who eat slowly. They feel they're missing all the fun playing outside with the children who wolfed down their lunch in a few moments. If your preschooler has this problem, discuss it with the teacher, who should allow your child more time to eat. Toddlers who wait too long for meals often lose their appetites altogether, so don't hold a hungry child off until the rest of the family is ready to eat. Since most children thrive on regularity, try to serve your toddler his or her meals and snacks at roughly the same time each day. Nutritional snacking, or better timed meals may be the answer.

Consistency, color, and texture of foods become increasingly important to the toddler, but just as important is not giving up feeding a particular food after a rejection. Some babies adapt slowly to new situations throughout life, and children with this inborn temperament often reject anything new, including new foods. This behavior fortunately can be modified once you understand that you have such a child. Keep re-introducing these rejected foods daily for about 20 days in a row. As familiarity develops, more often than not, your child will accept the food. **The single biggest error a parent makes in food introduction is giving up after a few tries.** On the other hand, it is important not to force the baby to eat a particular food. Just keep presenting the food daily until it is accepted. Keep feeding time happy and relaxed. Good nutrition can easily break down at this point if the parent gives up and offers the child a special diet of crackers, grapes, raisins , peanut butter, and juice. A parent may believe that this diet is "better than nothing." What follows is a fight of wills, and the "persistent child" rules! Instead, keep eating time a happy time. If your child is not interested in the nutritious foods you prepare, allow him to leave the table to play. Save his dish of uneaten food for the time when he might be hungrier, but don't give him any other food. There are a few other "don'ts" as well. Don't bargain with your child or promise "a dessert" after he finishes his plate. Many studies have confirmed that this method often makes things worse. The slow to adapt, persistent child subsequently remembers the treat and a negative pattern of behavior quickly develops. Remember that the baby is rejecting the food and not your love. This confusion can easily creep into your feelings and cause frustration and anger. Your child may have the persistence, but not the judgment to make adult decisions. **Never forget who the adult is!** If you judge that a particular food is not good for your child, don't offer it as a bribe or reward and certainly not as standard fare.

Don't forget the effect of stress on your child's appetite. Stress of all kinds may have an effect on appetite: parental pressure to eat, divorce, separation, illness within the family, job loss, a new baby, new child care arrangement, a new school, a new home or even an overly ambitious schedule can interfere with a child's appetite. Of course when a child is ill, one of the first things that happens is a decreased appetite. Unless it is a chronic illness, the appetite usually returns in about a week.

Try some of these food ideas on your baby:

Soups with peas, carrots, small pieces of meat or chicken, brown rice, potato or noodles. Children who get introduced to soups at 8-9 months of age continue to like it when textures change from smooth to lumpy. Some babies gag on lumpy food until they are older and this is normal. Don't be in a hurry to advance textures too early. Avoid putting high salt food into the soup such as ham or sausage. The child will not miss it, but if the baby already is used to salt, the soup might be rejected at first. As stated above, don't give up. Remember the twenty times rule! Appear indifferent to any rejections and don't make a fuss over rejected foods. It usually makes things worse.

(I suggest that you avoid serving Ramen noodles. They are extremely unhealthy because they are made by frying the noodles in saturated fat before drying. Top Ramen along with most instant cup of soups should be avoided at any age. Their high sodium and fat content make these easy to prepare items a poor choice for snack or lunch.)

Here are a few other suggestions for easy to prepare, nutritious finger foods, that make excellent snacks:

Soft sweet peas
Soft cooked carrot cubes
Small pieces of very ripe banana
Firm pieces of egg white or scrambled eggs
Brown rice or small pieces of boiled potato (no French fries)
Small pieces of poached or baked salmon or white fish, such as tilapia
Small pieces of boiled or baked chicken (Skin removed).

MORE ON PICKY EATERS

Parents love "good eaters." They give back so much pleasure and that wonderful feeling of successful parenting. Mothers dream of the baby whose mouth is always ready for another morsel of "love." Then there is the nightmare baby who resists all initial attempts at being fed. These children can often be identified shortly after birth. As described above, they quickly undermine the confidence of the most secure parent! It is to the parent of such a child that I am addressing the following paragraph. It's not too late to undo poor eating habits.

Most toddlers eat less than they did the first year of life and sometimes refuse meals completely. A toddler is not growing as fast as he was during his first year, therefore his caloric needs are less. He or she still requires nutritious foods, but less. The slow to adapt, persistent toddler now seems to be living on air. Mothers panic and conclude, "Better to give the child something—anything–rather than nothing." So eventually the toddler's diet is reduced to several glasses of juice a day plus crackers, cookies, peanut butter, raisins and grapes. Most crackers and chips have an outrageous ratio of calories from saturated fat and more salt than is healthy. About half the calories in Triscuits, Wheat Thins, Ritz Crackers , and Pepperidge Farms Goldfish come from fat. The result is a skinny and extremely cranky child. It's raisins in and raisins out (in the B.M.) minus what sticks to the teeth, causing early decay. Real fresh squeezed juice is essentially pure sugar water which further destroys the child's appetite and decays the teeth. Add grapes and crackers and you have one of the worst possible diets for a child. Of course the child will hold out for these "foods"; however the persistent, slow to adapt child will eventually respond to your efforts.

Here's the cure. Immediately stop ALL juice, raisins, crackers, cookies, peanut butter-jelly sandwiches and grapes! Remove all chips, Fritos, etc. from the kitchen cabinet.[33] In two to three days your child will be eating and drinking milk and wholesome foods again–as long as there are no other choices. The traditional advice found in most parenting books just doesn't work on children with this temperament. Try your best not to show frustration. **Be gentle, but firm** in not returning to the old diet. After your toddler is back on track, limit juice to only once a day and in a cup rather than in a bottle. If the child is thirsty offer

[33] The most common complaint that I hear from the mother is, "But my husband or boyfriend insists on having such junk foods around plus ice cream in the freezer!"

plain water (unsweetened). The rule of thumb is, "all favorite liquids go in a cup and only water in the bottle."

ADVICE ON HOW TO GENTLY BREAK THE BOTTLE AND PACIFIER HABIT

Many parenting books recommend that a child's bottle be removed at one year to prevent tooth decay. A child may tote a bottle filled with juice (which is essentially sugar water) or milk all day and night. For those parents who feel the baby "needs" the bottle, it would be wise for them to put only water (never diluted juice) in the bottle and all "good" things, such as milk, go into a cup. This will make it easier for you to remove the bottle in the future when you feel **you** can handle the change. Here is one method of change to a cup that I have employed successfully over many years. It is virtually painless for the child and parent.

When the child is between fifteen to eighteen months old, put only water in the bottle as described above. After a week or two, tell your child that the "Bottle Man" is coming on Saturday to get all the bottles and pacifiers to give to the little babies. Even if you think the baby will not understand what you are saying, it is important that you repeat this message with a happy and enthusiastic voice. Saturday morning, **before breakfast,** collect all the bottles, nipples, caps **and pacifiers with your child and have him put them in a large paper shopping bag.** Together, place the bag contents outside your front door and remind him **in a happy and enthusiastic voice** that the bottle man will be there to get these items for the little babies. Next, eat breakfast together. **After breakfast** remind your child about the bag and investigate to see whether the **Bottle Man** came. The bag should be empty of the bottles, but inside he should find a **new Teddy Bear,** or similar stuffed animal. Toy cars, trucks or other items do not work as well as a stuffed animal. Explain that this is a present from the **Bottle Man**. Now the child can **substitute this stuffed animal for the bottle** as a security item and also cuddle it at bedtime. Instead of giving him a bottle at bedtime, cuddle your child in your lap and continue your bedtime ritual using a cup. **Once you make the conversion it is extremely important not to return to the bottle**. If he asks for the bottle or pacifier, **remind him that the Bottle Man gave them to the little babies, and give him the stuffed doll that the Bottle Man left for him or her!** Do not attempt the conversion when your child is ill. Using this method, weekends are an ideal time to convert to a cup. The most common comment I get from parents is, **"Had I known it would be so easy I'd have done it sooner!"**

My daughter called me recently, concerned that her two-year-old was too skinny. She asked if there were some vitamin, mineral supplement or magic tonic that would boost his appetite. She was sure I would know what it was. Fortunately, I had kept her health records from the time she was a baby, and I faxed her the pertinent information. Her height-weight proportions were almost exactly the same as her at the same age. He was doing just fine. Inappropriate expectations can cause much anxiety in a parent. Remember that genetic factors and matters of temperament will also have something to do with how robust an eater your child will become.

Eating disorders often begin with the too-skinny two-year-old child whose parents make food the center of his existence. If your child refuses to eat as much as usual for more than a few days, don't be alarmed. This is often normal. The most common cause of a decrease in appetite is illness or a cold. Once the cold is over the appetite returns. Consult with your doctor if your child's appetite remains poor. But if your toddler looks well proportioned in spite of his "poor appetite" perhaps your expectations of how much food he needs is in error.

Several years ago a foster parent called me because she believed her two and a half year old had emotional problems.

She thought the cause might be the family's forthcoming move to a new community. The child was no doubt insecure, she said, though he needn't be. The problem was his stealing food - from their plates at mealtime, and by slipping out of bed to raid the refrigerator in the middle of the night. The child was bloated from overeating, the foster mother told me, even though she had cut back on his regular meals in order to compensate for the extra food he was sneaking.

Your guess is correct. The little boy was starving. By the time I saw him he was emaciated.

Although this is an extreme case, it demonstrates how errors in nutritional assessment can be made - even by educated, well-meaning people. These foster parents were both college graduates; the father was a minister. I'm convinced that neither of them would have purposefully done harm to the child they were raising. But our perceptions are clouded by personal bias as well as inexperience. For this reason it's important to check in with your child's physician periodically to ensure that the child's weight and development are within normal ranges.

Well-child checks are designed to spot early problems and provide guidance - both important facets of preventive health care. It's a myth that left to their own choices, children will naturally select the food they need over a period of time. Most children in our culture gravitate toward the worst junk foods and some of the most potentially harmful non-nutritious snacks.

We can't really expect our kids, especially the very young ones, to resist fast food advertising propaganda, peer pressure, and vending machines. <u>We</u> haven't resisted.

But we must. Now's the time to get our nutritional house in order, even in the face of the most convincing pleas. Trust me. As the father of five, I've heard some pretty compelling reasons for buying Sugar Frosted Flakes, potato chips, and beef jerky.

As stated earlier, don't use food as a reward, and don't withhold food as a punishment. Give a toy, watch a video together, or take a trip to the zoo as recognition for your child's achievement

- for having put away his toys, for doing well in school. Avoid making "treat" synonymous with food or sweets.

Keep mealtimes pleasant and relaxed. Traditionally, the family gathers together at mealtime. In our culture we usually meet at the end of the day. This is a time to share our day's experience and what was nice about the day. This may not be the best time to discuss the disaster at school or frustration at work. Work on accentuating the positive when food is served. (And turn off the TV during mealtimes!)

You will be getting much advice on what type of milk to give to your child. A fuss is being made over giving whole milk to your child until he or she is over two years old before introducing low fat milk. The truth of the matter is that 2% milk contains adequate fat for optimal brain growth and is the preferred type of milk for children between one and two. When children eat whole grains, vegetables and meat too, they get a more than sufficient amount of fat for optimal growth and nutrition. One percent low fat milk is probably also fine for most children as well, but I usually reserve this for children approaching two. The transition to non-fat milk is gradually made after two years of age. I'm not aware of a single case of nutritional problems due to "too little fat" in children over a year old that followed this advice. If you have a child who is exceptionally thin, it is important that you consult your pediatrician or health care provider to re-evaluate your child's diet and health. A complete history and physical examination is needed. Don't attempt to "fatten the child up" with high saturated fat foods.

SNACKS

When my son was born he quickly adapted to an every-two-hours eating schedule. My wife kept asking me when this demanding schedule would change. Twenty - five years later she notes that it never has changed: he has breakfast, a mid-morning snack, lunch, and afternoon snack, dinner, and a snack before bed. His "grazing" six or more meals a day did not make him overweight. **Calories do count,** but his total calorie intake over 24 hours was sufficient to cover what he burned from activity plus his growth needs.

Eating between meals gets bad press, but I think this is more about **what** we eat than **when** we eat. The human digestive tract is especially well adapted to snack-type eating rather than three major meals a day. As long as what we're eating is low in percentage of calories from fat, low in salt and not totally without fiber as a result of consuming ultra refined snacks, nibbling throughout the day is no problem.

The problem is that many nibble-type foods are high in saturated fat, high in salt, and low in fiber. Potato chips, corn chips (even "health food store" chips), granola bars, trail mix, crackers, cookies, doughnuts, cupcakes, ice cream, peanut butter and jelly, soda, Kool Aid, Hi-C, juice, milk shakes, salted nuts, and a variety of candy bars, are examples. **Health food stores, drugstores and supermarkets line their shelves with power bars, energy bars and snack bars that are essentially candy bars, marketed with unsubstantiated claims that these candy bars are healthy snacks made with an "ideal ratio" of simple to complex carbohydrates, along with protein and fat. There is no proof that such an ideal ratio exists!**

The "staying power" of the "instant energy" sports or chocolate bars are platitudes invented by copy-writers.

Lighter Bake[34] can be used as a substitute for fat in many baked goods.

---

[34] **Life is a compromise. Baked goods need not be high in fat. Sunsweet's Lighter Bake*** is a fat-free, fruit based replacement for butter or oil in recipes. Baked goods made with Lighter Bake instead of regular high trans-fat shortening have 10-30% fewer calories and 50-90% less fat. For each cup of oil, substitute 1/2 cup of **a** blend of apples and prunes.

Snacking is good. Don't change the habit, change the choice of your snacks.

PRESCHOOLERS: SNACKS

Children like simple snacks. Frozen bananas are a favorite treat for the two-year-old and older. Peel any overripe bananas, those with dark skins that you usually discard. Cut them in half, then place each half in a plastic Zip-Lock bag and freeze. Once frozen, simply serve - no preparation is required.

Whole wheat bagel and non-fat or 1% cream cheese is another favorite. Don't forget cut-up fresh fruit, corn kernels, peas, or garbanzo beans. Hummus[35] is made by blending chick peas (garbanzos), adding a few drops of lemon, and blending in favorite non-salt spices that the child likes. This is a more nutritious substitute for peanut butter or cream cheese. Another favorite is low fat, low salt vegetarian chili beans, prepared from scratch or from a can. Health Valley makes delicious, wholesome chili. Matzo and water crackers are good choices with low sodium mozzarella string cheese. A whole wheat English muffin with low salt tomato sauce and a slice of mozzarella cheese, microwaved, makes an instant pizza snack. Small cut-up pieces of chicken breast, or for the older child, a baked chicken leg, sprinkled with paprika and served over a bowl of brown rice make an excellent school lunch, transported in a Tupperware-like container. Air popped pop-corn is an excellent choice for children over five years old. **Younger children should avoid pop corn because it is easy to choke on**. Smoothies, especially on warm days, made with non-fat milk and seasonal fruit are nutritious and loved by most children, but not too often!

---

[35] There are many excellent commercially prepared brands of hummus available at most grocery stores.

THE TRUTH ABOUT PEANUT BUTTER

Peanuts are one of the most allergenic foods. Peanut butter can act like a plaster patch on the back of a very young child's throat to block the airway. My dentist used to say that peanut butter was the plaster that attaches sugar to teeth (jelly being 100 % sugar).

Peanut butter has a reputation for being a super source of protein. Four level tablespoons of peanut butter can provide your 7-10 year old with 16 grams of protein or half the protein he needs in a day. (The RDA for protein for a child 7-10 years old is 28 grams.) However, those four tablespoons contain a whopping 32 grams of fat[36] and 400 calories. Seventy five percent of those calories come from fat! Commercial peanut butter such as Skippy or Jif uses additional hydrogenated fat - usually hydrogenated cottonseed oil to improve spreading and prevent the peanut oil from separating. Cottonseed oil originates from the cotton plant, which has probably been sprayed with pesticide, thus endowing the oil with trace pesticidal properties. Salt and sugar are also added to commercial peanut butter to prevent mold growth and separation of the oil-fats such as butter or fats high in trans-fat ("hydrogenated"fats). As noted above though, peanut butter contains many other ingredients to make it less of an ideal food for children and adults.

And that's not all. Peanuts contain aflatoxin, a naturally occurring carcinogen and liver toxin that is produced by mold on damp peanuts. Roasting does not destroy this heavy duty toxin. The U.S. Department of Agriculture has a good program in place to minimize aflatoxin contamination of peanuts in commercially processed peanut butters and it seems to be keeping contamination down to acceptably low levels. "Real" peanut butter, made from ground peanuts in a home processor or at the health food store is believed to have ten times the amount of aflatoxin as the Skippy or Jif type brands.

---

[36] Peanut butter is high in total fat, but monounsaturated fat is the predominant type of fat. Nutritionists argue that monounsaturated fats may actually be good for you. That is why peanut oil is preferred over saturated fats

Don't be fooled by a label that claims "No Cholesterol Food!" Remember that cholesterol isn't found in any vegetable fat. Be aware that "reduced fat" peanut butter is still not low fat though it may contain a fourth less fat. To produce the "reduced fat" peanut butter, the manufacturer replaces about a quarter of the peanuts with soy protein. But then the product can't be called peanut butter anymore. It becomes a "spread."

Peanut butter can be eaten occasionally, perhaps once a week in conservative amounts, but the daily peanut butter and jelly sandwich has got to go.

When you make a peanut butter sandwich, here are a few hints on how to lower its high calorie fat content:

1. Reduce the peanut butter to 1 tablespoon.
2. Substitute a thinly sliced or mashed ripe medium banana for the jelly.

This will produce a sandwich with 248 calories and 10 grams of fat or 32 % of calories coming from fat.

Study the following statistics[37] before preparing your child's next peanut butter sandwich!

- ▲ **The odds of winning California's SuperLotto jackpot are 1 in 18 million. The odds of some other events:**
- ▲ **1 in 1 million (18 times more likely) to die from flesh-eating bacteria.**
- ▲ **1 in 650,000 (nearly 28 times more likely) to be killed by terrorists while traveling abroad.**
- ▲ **1 in nearly 650,000 to be dealt a royal flush on the opening hand in a poker game.**
- ▲ **1 in 48,000 (375 times more likely) to die of heart disease from eating a broiled steak a week.**
- ▲ **1 in 5000 (3,600 times more likely) to die of cancer from eating a daily peanut butter sandwich.**

[37] *Source: James Walsh, "True Odds," Merritt Publishing. 1996.

Try using Hummus as a substitute for peanut butter.

CHESTNUTS

A forgotten snack food is the **chestnut.** Chestnuts are high in complex carbohydrates, and contain a mere trace of fat - two large chestnuts have less than 30 calories and only 0.2 mg of fat.

I have fond memories of street vendors roasting chestnuts over charcoal fires on cold winter afternoons and evenings. This was in Innsbruck, Austria, in the 1950's, where I attended the University of Innsbruck when I wasn't skiing! The smell of roasted chestnuts sold them. We bought them in small bags, and the process of peeling away the shell and inner skin warmed frozen fingers.

Chestnuts are also good boiled and served with Brussels sprouts, or mashed and seasoned alongside small portions of lean roast meats. Introduce your family to chestnuts. It's a great snack food.

COOKING TIP: Try making the CHESTNUT STUFFING found in the Recipe Section.

A great way to introduce vegetables to young children is the recipe for LENTIL SOUP.

BASIC FOODS

When your child is between the ages of one and two, introduce (and reintroduce, if necessary) some basic foods: potato, corn, wheat, quinoa, and other grains, legumes and cruciferous vegetables, such as broccoli or Brussels sprouts. Be sure to include these on your plate which will make them appear more enticing to your youngster.

Potatoes, corn, wheat, grains, legumes and vegetables are important complex carbohydrates. Most contain significant protein and little fat (as long as they're not doused with butter, margarine, oil, or cream), as well as starch and fiber. These basic foods should be at the heart of your toddler's expanding diet. (See Chapter on carbohydrates for more information.)

FOOD FACT: Beans, Grains, and Vegetables are Basic Foods for children over age one. Tofu is also good to try. Read Chapter 4, and try the recipes for LENTIL SOUP, bean cuisine's "thick as fog split pea soup," black-eyed peas, bean dip, bean, turkey, and broccoli dinner, frijoles, basic mashed potatoes, baked potato, new potato with dill sauce, potato latkes (pancakes), organic tricolor quinoa, meat, brown rice, and ketchup, polenta, Veracruzana sauce, special cream of wheat, buckwheat pancakes, quick oatmeal, kasha varnishkas, millet pilaf, basic barley, broccoli, coleslaw, steamed vegetables, stir-fried vegetables, vegetable soup, vegetable sauté, green salad with vegetables, Hungarian butter lettuce salad, Hungarian cucumbers, carol's banana-strawberry smoothie, baked apple, apple sauce, peach sherbet, and baked pears French style in the recipe section.

THE FOODS CHILDREN NEED PART 1

▲ ▲ ▲

EGGS

Unless your child has eczema or has already shown an allergy to eggs, this food may safely be introduced to a child over age one or earlier in many cultures.

The egg is composed of egg white, one of the purest and best proteins available, and the egg yolk, a repository for cholesterol. Interestingly, people with already high cholesterol levels (over 200mg) don't experience much of an increase in their blood cholesterol level by eating eggs, whereas people with normal blood cholesterol (125-165mg) show a dramatic increase in cholesterol when they eat eggs.

Infants may need diets higher in cholesterol and fats than adults, but this should not be interpreted to mean that you must go out of your way to introduce high fat or high cholesterol foods.

Egg yolk has traditionally been introduced to children early because it had the reputation of being a great source of iron. But now we know that the iron in egg yolk is poorly absorbed by the body. I'm especially wary of large amounts of egg yolk because environmental poisons such as pesticide residues, which contaminate animal feeds, may show up in concentrated amounts in animal organs such as liver, eggs, and chicken skin.

On the other hand, egg white is an excellent non-fat uncontaminated source of protein. Boil an egg. Pop out the yolk and discard it. Chop up the white to garnish the salads of the older child. One to three eggs a week for a young child are nutritionally wholesome as long as they are not fried or prepared with butter or margarine.

FERTILE AND UNGRADED EGGS

A belief in **"vitalism"** prompts some people to buy fertilized eggs. From a nutritional point of view, fertilized and unfertilized eggs are identical. **The more important issue is that raw fertile eggs are a dangerous threat to health.** Graded eggs are sanitized using an antiseptic wash. Fecal germs on egg shells that haven't been through the antiseptic process cause hundreds of cases of food poisoning a year in the United States. Symptoms of salmonella food poisoning, which include nausea, vomiting, diarrhea, abdominal cramps, chills, fever, and achy muscles, usually begin 12-24 hours after eating contaminated food. Children, the elderly, and anyone with a compromised immune system are especially vulnerable to food poisoning.

Cartons of eggs sold in most supermarkets generally meet USDA Grade-A requirements. To be certain **never use raw or uncooked eggs. Even graded eggs are often contaminated. It is dangerous to put any raw egg in a "milkshake." Unpasteurized eggnog or Caesar salad dressing are extremely risky and should be avoided.**

COOKING TIP: Try the recipes for BASIC OMELETS, LOUIS'S DRENCH TOAST, and SCRAMBLED EGGS WRAPPED IN A TORTILLA found in the Recipe Section

TOFU

Tofu is a non-meat, non-dairy source of protein that is relatively high in calcium and low in price. It has been an important part of the Asian diet for more than 2000 years. Today most supermarkets and health food stores carry it. It's prepared from soybeans that have been soaked overnight, ground, boiled, strained, made into curd, cut into blocks, and kept refrigerated. Three-and-a-half ounces, or about 1/2 cup, contain about 145 calories and 8-10 grams of protein. Furthermore, soybean is a complete protein, that is, it contains all the essential amino acids. Although 3-1/2 oz. of tofu contain 9 grams of fat, it is cholesterol free and the fat is mostly polyunsaturated.

Tofu can be added to soup and salads, or barbecued. It can be stir-fried, broiled, grilled, sautéed, or baked. It can be pureed to make dips, spreads, salad dressing and when mashed, it can be substituted for ricotta or cottage cheese.

There are two basic types of tofu, soft and firm. Soft tofu comes in thick, straight-edged blocks; the firm type has compressed edges. When you buy tofu, check the date for freshness. Rinse the tofu when you get it home, place it in a container of fresh cold water, and store it in the refrigerator. Change the water daily.

Miso is another soy product. It is a salty seasoning paste made from a combination of soybeans and a grain such as rice or barley. This product should be avoided because its sodium content can exceed 900 milligrams per tablespoon.

POTATO

Along with rice, corn, and wheat, the potato is known worldwide as a staff of life. Spanish conquistadors carried it to Europe from the Andes in the 16th century, and it has become one of the most nutritious and versatile food staples.

It's a wonderful food, not at all fattening: a medium-size potato contains only 100 calories, is 99.9% fat free, and provides about half the Vitamin C a person needs in a day. Potato skin is high in dietary fiber and contains most of the Vitamin C. Although the potato isn't particularly rich in protein, its biological quality is as high or higher than the soybean protein.

People associate the Irish with potatoes, but I think of eastern Europe. My mother prepared potato soup, boiled potatoes, baked potatoes, and mashed potatoes. Remembering her potato latkes, potato kugel, and potato knadel still makes my mouth water. By the time of her death at age 94, she had supplied me with a generous variety of traditional Jewish potato recipes, some of which I've reprinted here, modified in the interest of less salt and fat.

Sadly, Americans have veered away from the wholesome use of potatoes. More than half of the potatoes we eat these days are in the form of potato chips, processed frozen French fries, fast-food French fries, and dehydrated potato preparations. In 1980, Americans ate five billion pounds of French fries, and one billion pounds of potato chips. While an 8-ounce potato has 140 calories, 8 ounces of potato chips contain 1200 calories, 28 teaspoons-full (133 grams) of which are pure fat!

While you still have some say in the matter, avoid starting your toddler on these foods. Stick to something wholesome such as my mother's basic mashed potatoes. But beware! Potato rapidly breaks down in the body to sugar, and for the anti-sugar advocates, this food is on their list of "forbidden fruit."

COOKING TIP: Try the recipes for BASIC MASHED POTATOES, BAKED POTATO, NEW POTATO WITH DILL SAUCE, and POTATO LATKES (PANCAKES) found in the Recipe Section.

RICE[38]

Rice is one of the most nutritious grains. It is the principal food for many millions of people throughout the world. Most children quickly learn to love rice. Although it doesn't contain an unusually high percentage of protein, it is of higher biological value[39] than corn. One half cup of rice contains about three grams of protein. Unpolished rice, such as brown rice, contains bran, a dietary fiber, in its husk. The husk is now being studied to see if it contains any anti-diabetes factors. Rice bran lowers blood cholesterol as much as oat bran, but unlike oat bran, rice bran doesn't turn gummy when cooked. You can buy rice bran which is packaged as wheat germ and is used is similar ways. Sprinkle it on cereal, salad, and non-fat yogurt, or add it to baked goods. An

38 Levels of lead in rice could pose a risk to children. April 12, 2013 US Scientists reported at an American Chemical Society meeting in New Orleans that researchers from Monmouth University in New Jersey found high levels of lead in our rice supply, especially from Bhtan, Italy, India and Thailand. Lead is a neurotoxin: it damages the brain, and in young children whose brains are still growing, can seriously diminish their capacity to learn and develop intellectually. There is also evidence that lead can disrupt children's behavior, such as make them more aggressive, impulsive and hyperactive. Although this information from Monmouth University has not been repeated or confirmed to date, be sure to following this research.

39 Protein foods have been classified according to their ability to be digested and used by the body. The measurement is called biological value. Egg white is considered to have the protein of highest known biological value. Following egg white, in descending order, are fish, cow milk, and cheese, brown rice, red meat, and poultry (Garrison and Somer, *Nutrition Desk Reference*, Keats Publishing, 1985).

ounce contains 8 grams of dietary fiber, 4 grams of protein, and lots of niacin, thiamin, magnesium, and iron.

In the 1890's there was a strange outbreak of an illness called beriberi in Asia characterized by fatigue, weight loss, emotional disturbances, impaired sensory perception, weakness and pain in the limbs, swelling of the body tissues, staggering gait, heart failure and death. To study this illness, some of the best physicians in the world were sent to study it. Dr. Christiaan Eijkman, a Dutch physician was sent to Indonesia to study this illness. He lived in a home to study a family with these symptoms. This home had a yard with chickens and goats as did many homes at that time. The diet of the family was mostly polished rice. Polished rice was developed, not because of its taste, but because brown rice has a short shelf life, while polished rice has a very long shelf life. One day the family ran out of the regular chicken feed usually used. Instead, the family began feeding their left over white rice to the chickens. Soon Dr. Eijkman noticed that the chickens began to become very aggressive and developed poor balance, stumbling and soon dying, similar to the family's beriberi.

Dr.Eijkman decided to feed the chickens unpolished brown rice. The chickens recovered! This was a "nutritional disease" and it was cured by consuming the unprocessed rice containing husks. The husk contained an anti-beriberi factor. This is how thiamine or vitamin B-1 was discovered. Dr. Eijkman was awarded the Nobel Prize.

Most of this had been forgotten because white rice was "enriched" with vitamins and beriberi became almost an historical illness.

Now there is an epidemic of diabetes mellitus in Asia, as it is in the USA. But the difference is that in India, Indonesia, the Philippines, Vietnam and China, the illness is not necessarily associated with obesity, as it is in the USA.

Recalling the beriberi epidemic, scientists once again began studying polished rice and found that those who consumed large amounts of rice 5 times a week were at high risk for developing diabetes mellitus while those who consumed brown rice had over 15% lower risk for developing it. Brown rice appears to be protective. If the white rice was substituted with whole grains, including brown rice, this was associated with a 35% lower diabetes risk. These data support the recommendation that most carbohydrate intake should come from whole unrefined grains.

FORMS OF RICE[40]

Short and medium grain rice is wetter than long rice and their kernels stick together. You can overcome the stickiness by adding oil to the water in which you cook the rice, but by now you know I wouldn't recommend any such thing. Don't add salt, either. If you don't like sticky rice, use long grain or parboiled rice.

Long grain rice is generally preferred for Chinese cooking and is good for curries, pilaf, or stews served over rice. The stickier rice is especially good for puddings or molded rice dishes, California roll sushi, and many Japanese dishes.

Kernels that break during the milling process are sold as **"broken rice,"** which is a little less expensive than other rice.

Whole grain rice, as opposed to **polished rice,** retains all the grain's nutrients, most notably vitamins and minerals otherwise lost in milling when the outermost husk is removed. **Brown whole grain rice** is a popular favorite. It has a nice nut-like flavor and is chewier than white rice. Short grain brown rice is even chewier than the long grain version.

Polishing or processing rice, as stated earlier, involves removing the outer layer. Polished rice has been discredited because it is deficient in B vitamins. Polished rice has a lower fat content than brown rice, so it is less likely to become rancid. This is the reason for the popularity of white rice-increased shelf life. Sup-

40

posedly polished rice also creates less gas in the bowels because it has less bran than the whole grain.

Enriched rice is polished rice to which iron, thiamine, and niacin have been returned in amounts approximately that of un-milled kernels. Uncle Ben's is a popular, easy to prepare "enriched" rice. You get the three B-vitamins and iron that are added to all enriched grains, but you lose the fiber, magnesium, vitamins E and B-6, copper, zinc, and other nutrients such as the poorly understood phytochemicals (plant chemicals) that are in the whole grains, such as brown rice.

Parboiled or **converted white rice** has been specially treated to retain vitamins. It may contain two to four times as much thiamine and niacin as polished white rice. The term "parboiled" is slightly misleading; the rice is not precooked, but is actually somewhat harder than regular rice. It takes a little longer to cook than regular white rice, but the grains will be very fluffy and separate after they have been cooked. My personal favorites are long grain brown rice and converted rice.

Precooked rice has been fully cooked and dehydrated after milling. This is the "instant" or "minute rice" that needs no preparation beyond pouring boiling water over the rice according to the package directions, and letting stand for a few minutes before serving. This stuff is pretty tasteless and less nutritious than other rice. The newest addition to instant rice is precooked converted rice that has been vacuum-packed in a plastic bag. Simply immerse it in boiling water as directed on the package and in a few moments you have perfectly prepared rice.

Arborio is a starchy white rice with an almost round grain. This is the rice used to make the Italian dish risotto and it also works well for paella and rice pudding. Arborio absorbs up to five times its weight in liquid as it cooks, which results in grains of a creamy consistency.

Wild rice is botanically unrelated to rice. It is a native grain to North America. Like rice, it grows in marshy land. French explorers found it growing around the Great Lakes and called it "crazy oats," although it is no more related to oats than to rice. Because it is difficult to produce in large quantities, wild rice is extremely expensive. It has a distinct nutty flavor and chewiness.

COOKING TIP: Try the recipe for MEAT, BROWN RICE, AND KETCHUP

CORN, WHEAT, QUINOA, AND OTHER GRAINS

Technically a grass, corn is the only cereal born and bred in America. It was the main food of the Indian civilizations of the Americas from the Canadian border to the Andes. The Pilgrims from England who settled here learned from the natives how to use corn.

The dried corn kernel is strong and hard on the outside, while its germ, or inside, is soft and almost floury. Indians showed the Southern Colonists how to pound, grind, and boil whole kernels in lye or lime water to make hominy, which remains a staple in the Southern diet. "Grits" refers to the flint-like, grainy, textured part of the kernel. (Unless cornmeal is soaked in water to soften it, the corn bread made from it is gritty.)

Toddlers tend to love corn bread, corn muffins, hominy grits, and corn flakes - all high in nutrients. Popcorn is one of the few popular snack foods that tastes good and provides solid food value, when not doused with butter, oil or salt as served in the Movie Theaters. **I don't recommend popcorn for children under five** because of the possibility of choking.

My favorite form of corn is on the cob. A few years ago I planted eight rows of Eastern white corn in our big backyard garden, but because I planted them all at the same time, we had five or six dozen ears of corn ready to be eaten all at the same time. Some farmer I turned out to be!

Our solution was a neighborhood "Pick Your Own" party and feast that was a huge success. It was the first time I had ever tried corn without butter or salt. It was fantastic!

If you buy fresh corn from a farmer's market, take along a cooler. Warm temperatures quickly convert the corn's sugar to starch. Select corn with plump, juicy, well aligned kernels that are tightly packed. Buy those ears of corn with the husks still on, and discard ears with rusty looking tips or shriveled kernels.

To steam sweet corn, heat it through for about 2-5 minutes. To grill, cut off tassels, remove the silk, leave the husks on and soak in ice water for 5 minutes. Place over the coals, a few inches from the fire's center. Turn every 5 minutes. In 15 minutes, the husk should be blackened and the corn ready to eat.

COOKING TIP: Try the recipes for POLENTA and VERA-CRUZANA SAUCE in the recipe section.

WHEAT

The most widely grown of all cereal grains, wheat is a kind of berry that consists of an outer covering, the bran, which is high in minerals, B vitamins, and some protein; and the inner part, or endosperm, which consists mainly of starch and protein. The wheat germ resides in the endosperm. The germ is comparatively high in fat and Vitamin E.

Wheat is made into white flour and whole wheat flour: White flour consists of ground endosperm only. Whole wheat or graham flour contains the bran and the entire endosperm. Because it contains the germ, which contains fat, whole wheat flour can spoil, whereas white flour can be stored fresh for much longer. On the other hand, whole wheat flour contains more fiber, minerals, vitamins, and slightly more protein than even enriched white flour (white flour to which thiamine, riboflavin, niacin, and iron have been added). Your toddler will enjoy whole wheat pasta, pilaf, and breads of many kinds. Bulgur wheat, very high in fiber, is made from several varieties of wheat. It is used as a cereal, in soups or salads, as a side dish or main meal. Too much can cause gassiness.

If your children have grown used to white bread, help them switch to whole wheat by preparing sandwiches with one slice of white and one slice of whole wheat bread. Another way to introduce whole wheat bread is to switch to a bread that looks like whole wheat but has the texture of white, such as Roman Meal. This will let your child adapt to the color of whole wheat over a couple of weeks or even a month. Then switch to a mild whole wheat bread. The older the child, the more slowly is the transition, especially with the slow to adapt, persistent child. Be patient and persistent. The long term gains are worth it.

COOKING TIP: Try the recipes for SPECIAL CREAM OF WHEAT and BUCKWHEAT PANCAKES.

RYE

Rye has a stronger, heartier flavor than wheat, and is typically used to make rye bread. Today's American rye bread is usually one-third rye flour, two-thirds whole wheat flour. When I was growing up it was the real thing, a traditional Jewish rye with caraway seeds and a crunchy crust. Onion and corn rye breads were my favorites. Authentic black pumpernickel, and German or Russian rye breads are also delicious, and you can find them in small local bakeries. They're worth hunting for.

Generally speaking, food from grains such as corn, wheat, or rye are among the most nutritious foods we eat (as long as we don't add butter or margarine).

For the five-year-old, try low or non-fat cheese, lettuce and **ripe tomato** sandwiches on rye, but hold the mayo.[41] Many children do not develop a taste for lettuce until four years of age, so don't be too upset if your toddler rejects salads. Keep trying, and be sure to make a salad a daily part of the adult diet. Remember, you're the role model!

OATS

Oats are an ancient grain, probably cultivated since the first century A.D. They are used most frequently as cattle food. Humans consume only about 5 % of the world oat crop. In America, oats are used mostly for hot cereal and more recently for muffins, cookies and breads. Oats are an excellent source of complex carbohydrate and contain about 50% more protein than bulgur wheat, and twice as much as brown rice. They are rich in vitamin E and the B vitamin, folate, as well as the minerals iron, copper, zinc and manganese. Oats are also a good source of dietary fiber, both soluble and insoluble. The soluble fiber is primarily responsible for lowering blood cholesterol. Two ounces of dry oats (1-1/3 cups cooked) contain 5 grams of fiber and only one gram of fat.

Granola is made from oats, but many commercial brands are extremely high in fat. Often highly saturated tropical oil, such as palm or coconut oil, is added to the oats before they are toasted. You can buy low fat granola or you can make your own. Toast quick or old-fashioned rolled oats on a baking sheet in a 300o F oven and stir frequently. If you wish, stir in honey[42] to taste before toasting. Be careful not to scorch. After toasting, mix in

[41] Some non-fat mayonnaise has such poor taste, you may want to return to your favorite high fat brand. Shop around and don't give up. There are improved and more tasty non-fat mayo-substitutes arriving weekly at your market.

[42] Do not give honey to infants under one year of age. Refer to earlier warnings concerning the danger of infant botulism from honey. It is safe to use honey after the baby is over one year old.

your choice of wheat germ, bran, and chopped dried fruits. Let cool in a plastic bag or refrigerator. Bear Naked, Peak Protein, and Tally Free Organic Granola are wholesome choices.

"Bear Naked" natural granola has only 0.5grams of saturated fat, the rest being the more healthy mono and polyunsaturated fat, zero cholesterol, 3 grams of dietary fiber, 6 grams of protein and only 6 grams (1-1/2 teaspoons sugar). No artificial flavors or artificial preservatives.

Muesli is a cold cereal, very popular in Switzerland, Germany and Austria. Like granola, mass-market muesli is often high in fat and calories, but you can prepare your own fairly easily. Mix uncooked rolled oats with rolled wheat flakes, bite-sized shredded wheat, wheat nuggets, 100% bran shreds, oat or wheat bran, or wheat germ. Stir in any of your favorite dried fruits and a small amount of unsalted, coarsely chopped nuts or seeds. If you prefer sweet muesli, add a little brown sugar, maple syrup, or molasses. Serve only to children over three or four, because younger children may choke on the seeds. Store in an airtight container in the refrigerator. If muesli is mixed with skim milk and refrigerated overnight, it will have the consistency of cooked cereal. If you prefer it crunchy, stir in non-fat milk or non-fat yogurt just before serving.

COOKING TIP: Try the recipe for QUICK OATMEAL

ETHNIC GRAINS

Buckwheat isn't related to wheat, and isn't even a cereal. Technically or botanically, it's a fruit. In any case, it's another wonderful complex carbohydrate around which to build a meal. In middle European countries, buckwheat groats, or kernels, are prepared similarly to rice and called **kasha.** It is necessary to roast the kasha before boiling as roasting keeps it from developing a sticky, porridge-like consistency. Kasha and yogurt is an ethnic favorite among Eastern European Jews, as is **"kasha varnishkas,"** kasha with bow-tie noodles. The kernels can also be processed into flour for pancakes or waffles.

Barley, sold whole or pearled (with the tough though nutritious bran covering removed), is another delicious complex carbohydrate that not many Americans know about. In this country barley is used more as a source of malt for beer production; but cooked with raisins and grated lemon peel, it makes a nutritious and delicious cereal high in fiber, iron and other nutrients. It's also good in casseroles and soups. Aside from the flavor, I love the chewy texture of this grain.

Millet is a term applied to a variety of small seeds used mainly for birdseed in this country, but in Africa, India, and China, millet is a staple grain. The most popular millets are sorghum, the premier cereal in Africa, used in the U.S. mostly for sorghum syrup; or pearl millet, which you can usually find in health food stores for use as a cereal, or in meal form. Millet is used to make porridge in North Africa and roti (a flat bread) in India.

Quinoa pronounced "keen-wah" is technically a seed, not a grain and is grown high in the Andes Mountains of South America. This pseudo-cereal is not a member of the true grass family. The nutrient composition is very good compared with common cereals. It is a good source of protein, fiber, calcium and is therefore a good food for vegans and those who are lactose intolerant. Quinoa contains no gluten or wheat.

It cooks very easily, in about 15 minutes. Cook it in a pot as you do rice. Cook it at a high setting until is starts boiling and then cover and simmer for about 12-15 minutes. Be careful not to use too much water otherwise it will take longer to cook. Stir the quinoa so all the water gets absorbed.

It can be used instead of pasta and served with marinara sauce over it. Additional recipes are found in the Recipe Section.

COOKING TIP: Try the recipes for KASHA VARNISHKAS, MILLET PILAF, and BASIC BARLEY

BEANS, PEAS, LENTILS, AND OTHER LEGUMES

Legumes are vegetables that come in pods. They include all beans, often named for their shape or color: kidney, black, pink, red, or white; peas, which are usually round but also grow elongated and multicolored such as black-eyed peas; and lentils, flat, disk-like legumes that are green or pink or orange, and are sold whole or split. The peanut is also a legume, not a nut.

White beans, red beans, kidney beans, black-eyed peas, lentils, and garbanzos are all similar in content - they are outstanding complex carbohydrates, low in fats and salt, and high in fiber. They are also very economical, and among the most nourishing of vegetables. Use them in casseroles and soups, in salads or as a side dish. They're also a good source of water-soluble vitamins, especially thiamine, riboflavin, niacin, and folate.

Red, white, and kidney beans, black-eyed peas, lentils, and garbanzos are generally packaged dried, and most are available canned or frozen. Dried peas and beans lose their nutritional value after about a year of storage. Frozen and canned beans usually contain too much salt, but canned no-salt added legumes are now showing up in most grocery stores.

Aside from highest grades for nutritional and economic value, beans are rich in anti-carcinogenic substances that may prevent or control certain cancers. Soybeans[43] contain a particular type of anti-carcinogen that may reduce the risk of some hormone-dependent cancers, such as breast or prostate.

"Beano" is sold in most grocery and health food stores as an aid to reduce gassiness. It is a digestive aid. When a couple of drops of this digestive enzyme is added to your first spoonful of beans or lentils, the result are like magic! It is very effective, practically tasteless, and safe. For those of you unable to tolerate legumes because of gassiness, I highly recommend this additive. It is also safe for toddlers. Follow the directions on the label.

COOKING TIP: Try the recipes for lentil soup, bean cuisine's "Thick as Fog split pea soup," Black-eyed Peas, Bean dip, Bean, Turkey, and Broccoli dinner, and Frijoles

YELLOW VEGETABLES

Yellow vegetables are rich in beta carotenes, which convert to Vitamin A when eaten. Carrots, squash, yams[44] or sweet potatoes

[43] The once lowly soybean was considered, until recently, to be good for nothing but animal feed. Now soybeans prepared as textured soy protein burgers and tofu has gone mainstream. The chemical, genistein, found in soybeans, first identified in 1987, is believed to be effective in preventing prostate cancer or slowing progression of early stage prostate cancer when combined with a high fiber, low animal fat diet. Because the phytoestrogens found in soy mimics real estrogen, some of the discomfort of menopause may be alleviated by women who consume soy products. That's the theory as to why a lot of Asian women experience less symptoms and hot flashes. They get a tremendous amount of soy and have all their lives.

[44] Yams or sweet potatoes are rich in fiber, complex carbohydrates, calcium, potassium, vitamin A and C. Despite the name, yams are related to the morning glory family and not the potato (from the Andes). When shopping for yams, choose smooth, hard tubers that are free of mushy spots, cuts or bruises. They should seem heavy for their size. Store yams in a cool, dry place, suspended in a wire basket or in an open paper (not plastic) bag. Do not refrigerate, which hardens the yam flesh and degrades its taste. Baked yams are

are examples of vegetables loaded with carotenes. Yellow corn and cantaloupe are also rich in Vitamin A or beta carotene. If you are looking for foods high in Vitamin A, think yellow.

Fortunately most children love carrots. The younger child should be given only steamed or cooked carrots because raw carrots may cause choking. For the older child, however, carrots make a wonderful snack. Supermarkets now sell ready prepared, peeled small carrots in bags. With the exception of beets, carrots contain more sugar than any other vegetable, which explains why children find it to be a satisfying snack eaten raw and a tasty addition to a variety of cooked dishes.

TOMATOES

Tomatoes complement many other foods such as poultry, meats, fish, pasta, pizza, and most other vegetables. Perhaps that is why it is one of the most popular vegetables among Americans. Botanically, the tomato is a fruit, but in 1893, the Supreme Court of the United States, in its wisdom, proclaimed it a vegetable! Whether tomatoes are a fruit or vegetable doesn't really matter; they are a delicious food, especially if grown in your garden.

At one time fresh ripe tomatoes were my favorite food. They were grown for flavor and I'd enjoy tomato sandwiches, tomato marinated with vinegar and onion, or tomato salad. Anything with tomato made a meal more delicious. Much of this has changed with the selection and cultivation of tomato varieties designed for shelf life, machine harvesting, size and shape for canning, with flavor being last on the scientist's plant design list. The university's plant science department has become an extension of agribusiness. These ubiquitous "cardboard" tomatoes should be avoided, and then industry might get the message that consumers desire flavor along with appearance. Greenhouse tomatoes are distinguished by the part of the stem and leaves still attached when they are sold. These are somewhat more tasty than those artificially ripened with ethylene gas on the way to the market. Try growing your own with your child this spring. The taste of a home grown tomato is a revelation! Next best: organic tomatoes at the Farmers Market. Children love to garden, and those who do are likely to taste and enjoy the fruits of their labor.

Tomatoes that are refrigerated or exposed to temperatures below 55oF lose their ripening potential. If you buy tomatoes slightly under-ripe, place them in a paper bag with an apple or banana and let them ripen at room temperature for a few days. This will enhance their flavor and texture.

When you buy canned tomato products such as tomato sauce, tomato puree, tomato paste, or stewed tomatoes, it is best to choose the "no salt added" brands. **The regular cans contain as much as twelve times the sodium of unsalted brands.** Avoid tomato juice and V-8 type juices which also contain an enormous amount of salt. Most cans were lined with the chemical BPA, but hopefully the replacement lining will turn out to be less harmful.

Many children develop a rash around the mouth from the peel oils found under the skin of tomatoes. This is due to irritation and is not allergy. To prevent rash, wash your child's face with warm water and a mild soap, such as Dove, to remove peel oil.

Tomatoes are rich in vitamin C, beta carotene, and potassium. They also contain some zinc, iron, folate, and the phytochemical[45] lycopene. Lycopene, an anti-oxidant carotenoid, and other tomato nutrients may reduce the risk of prostate cancer. Tomatoes may also reduce the risk of stroke in men by as much as 55%. That is because the ingredient linked to stroke protection is lycopene. The red color common to tomato, watermelon, grapefruit and guava signals lycopene (a plant pigment).

---

[45] Phytochemicals are substances isolated from fruit and vegetables that have medicinal power. They are considered to be non-nutritive because they aren't necessary for human growth, as are vitamins and minerals.

Lycopene is a potent antioxidant working in the body to counter free radicals that can damage cells and their DNA. This antioxidant may also reduce inflammation and cholesterol, prevent blood clots, and boost immune function. All studies were done on lycopene rich foods, not what Health Food Industry promotes as a pill. To obtain the benefits of lycopene, eat those foods high in lycopene such as tomato puree, Marinara sauce, tomato salsa, sun dried tomato, cooked tomato, tomato paste, raw tomato, cherry tomato, grapefruit, grapefruit, guava, and watermelon.

Vine-ripened tomatoes have a higher lycopene content than tomatoes ripened off the vine.

Every vegetable, every fruit, has hundreds of phytochemicals. This is one more reason to increase fruit and vegetable consumption.

The following are of no proven benefit for cardiovascular risk reduction: vitamin C, vitamin E. or beta-carotene supplementation; garlic; selenium; and chromium.

GREENS

Green vegetables range in color from light to dark. They can be used raw in salads, or cooked into interesting side dishes. They are high in Vitamin A (they contain beta carotene like yellow vegetables), Vitamin C, and folic acid or folate, and they contain significant amounts of calcium and iron. Along with other complex carbohydrates, they are an important component to the healthy diet.

Greens generally used in salads are the crispy iceberg and Romaine lettuces, and softer leaf lettuces, such as butter leaf, red leaf, oak leaf and others. The darker the greens, the more nutrition. Although iceberg lettuce is the number one best seller in the United States, it's the least nutritious variety of lettuce. Romaine and loose-leaf lettuces, for example red leaf, contain more vitamin A and calcium than iceberg. Butterhead varieties have more iron. Aside from lettuce, other delicious greens to add to a salad are endive, watercress, dandelion, spinach, Swiss chard, and mustard greens.

Greens good for cooking are mustard and beet greens, collard, kale, chard, and spinach. These also add tasty, colorful, textural interest to some casseroles.

Experiment with all these greens. Try the ones you've never tasted. You may discover you've been missing out on some delicious vegetables.

Green vegetables are the most common rejects of young children. If you keep preparing and eating them yourself, your youngsters will gradually accept them as part of the normal fare. Hopefully, the habit will continue into the teenage years, when the independent-minded child divorces himself from anything green and goes on a pizza, soda, potato chip, corn dog and M&M diet. If your family seldom eats green vegetables, it's never too late to correct poor eating choices and habits.

CRUCIFEROUS VEGETABLES

The name, cruciferous comes from the Latin word meaning "cross," because these vegetables bear cross-shaped flowers. Family members include cabbage, cauliflower, Brussels sprouts, watercress, broccoli, horseradish, kale, kohlrabi, mustard, radishes, rutabaga, turnip, Asian and collard greens. These vegetables contain cancer fighting compounds called *indoles*. Cruciferous vegetables seem to help protect against cancer of the stomach and large intestine. Studies strongly suggest that these vegetables stimulate the release of anti-cancer enzymes. These enzymes and the antioxidant nutrients, such as carotenoid (beta carotene and vitamin A) and vitamin C, help remove free radicals, unstable oxygen molecules that promote cancer. As a bonus, most cruciferous vegetables are good sources of dietary fiber. Kale, collard greens, and turnip greens also supply calcium, while others such as Brussels sprouts provide iron. Fortunately most children enjoy broccoli. Experiment with this group of vegetables[46]and introduce them early so your child will develop a taste for these wholesome foods.

COOKING TIP: Try the recipes for broccoli, coleslaw, steamed vegetables, stir-fried vegetables, vegetable soup, vegetable sauté, green salad with vegetables, Hungarian butter lettuce salad, and Hungarian cucumbers.

ONIONS

Onions rank sixth among the world's leading vegetable crops. They are cousins to garlic, leeks, chives, and shallots. Americans eat 50% more onions today than we did ten years ago. The bulbs now rank just behind potatoes and lettuce as our most popular vegetable. Many onions, such as Maui Sweet or red Bermudas, are quite juicy because of their high sugar content. Spanish onions are the largest and range in color from yellow to purple and have a mild flavor. White onions tend to be more pungent than yellows or reds. There are no nutritional differences among these types. Select onions that feel dry and solid all over, with no soft spots or sprouts. Avoid onions with green areas or a strong odor, which is a sign of decay. Cut raw onions produce volatile compounds that irritate the eyes. To lessen eye irritation, hold onions under cold running water as you peel. Chilling onions beforehand also helps.

Cooking onions produces a chemical change that makes them much milder. The heat convert's some compounds found in onions into a substance that is fifty to seventy times sweeter than table sugar! Although onions are not loaded with vitamins, they

[46] Offer these vegetables daily in a soup, in salad, as a snack with a dip, raw, steamed, stir fried, mixed with pasta, in tomato sauce or in a Spanish omelet.

contain antioxidants called phytochemicals, (plant chemicals), that in laboratory tests have blocked the earliest changes in cells that enable tumors to grow. These are mostly sulfur-containing compounds, or organosulfurs, the same ones that irritate your eyes and give onions their sharp taste. Onions also are reported to lower a blood pressure and cholesterol levels and may protect against stomach and esophageal cancers. They are a low-fat food and a great flavor enhancer for potatoes, rice, fish, ground meat, sandwiches, and soup. Virtually every cooking method has been used with onions; however avoid recipes that call for added fats. Also avoid fried onion rings which are extremely high in fat, as well as high fat onion cheese dips and French onion soup.

GARLIC

Garlic is a close relative of the onion. There is much hype about the medicinal powers of garlic, and health food stores continue to make claims that it protects the heart and is an anti-cancer food. To date, few trustworthy studies substantiate these claims. The National Cancer Institute and other universities are currently studying garlic and onion for such effects, but take heart, though: garlic wards off vampires![47]

Many Latin-American children are introduced to garlic at an early age. It is an excellent taste enhancer and you might want to experiment with it by making salad dressing with garlic vinegar. Place several peeled cloves in a bottle of wine vinegar and let stand for two to three days, covered, and then remove the garlic. Garlic or onion bread is another favorite. Heat the bread in the oven or microwave and then slice the loaf open. Rub the inside with a halved garlic clove or spread with baked garlic and then toast it under the broiler. If you want to use a mild olive oil or

[47] Dracula: Bram Stoker, 1897. "There are things that so afflict him that he has no power, as the garlic that we know of... "

Parmesan cheese on the bread, use sparingly. Avoid butter or margarine.

FRUIT

The most wonderful thing about fruit is that it is that children adore its sweetness, yet it is extremely healthy. Of course too much of any good thing isn't a good idea, so beware of the **fruitaholic**, the child who is on a total fruit diet, such as grapes, raisins, and juice! It is not the purpose of this book to review in depth all fruit, but I do want to give you an overview to help you understand why fruit is nutritionally important and should be a part of your child's daily diet.

With a few exceptions, such as avocado, fruit is nearly fat-free. Many fruits, especially apples, are high in cholesterol-lowering and blood-sugar stabilizing **fiber** and also supply some minerals. Three of the most popular fruits, bananas, pears, and oranges, are loaded with potassium, while berries and dried fruit are rich in iron. Citrus fruits, berries, kiwi and papaya are rich in vitamin C. Yellow and orange fruits such as apricots, cantaloupes, peaches, nectarines, and mangoes, are the best sources of beta carotene (vitamin A) and other carotenoids.[48]

Although grapes are usually not thought of as being especially nutritious, recently a cancer-preventing substance has been found in high concentrations in grapes. This suggests that there may be even more powerful compounds in other natural foods. This finding does not mean that people should eat a lot of grapes to prevent cancer. The overall message is that fruits and vegetables are very useful against disease.

Another health benefit of grapes,[49] *for adults,* comes from drinking wine, which can protect against heart attacks. In

[48] Read more about carotenoids in Part II - Vitamin A.

[49] Red grape juice appears to slow the activity of blood platelets, making

particular, red wine may protect against heart disease by preventing the formation of blood clots that can block arteries.

Don't forget that the whole grape is a common choking food and should not be given to toddlers *under two.*

There are few short cuts to good nutrition. Each week a new herbal, vitamin or mineral is featured at the health food store promising the consumer greater longevity, and a clearer, more facile mind. This approach is specifically derived from soft evidence suggesting some benefits from an amino acid, vitamin, mineral or herb and sold as a panacea. These products are very iffy at best. As an example, beta carotene taken as a supplement by smokers actually increased morbidity and mortality due to lung cancer instead of giving the assumed protection. I am not saying that supplements are not important. They definitely are. Especially vitamin D, vitamin C, folic acid, vitamin E, vitamin B-12, (especially in the elderly and vegan- vegetarians), B-6 in certain select groups, calcium and selenium. But there is little evidence that these nutrients help very much if the consumer consumes a balanced diet high in fiber, low in sodium and saturated fats.

To get the protective effect of these nutrients, you must eat adequate amounts of fruits and vegetables every day. Foods work together in concert. Isolating any of the many nutritional compounds and putting them in a pill form unfortunately causes them to lose most of their effectiveness for reasons that are not

---

them less likely to clot and cause heart attacks in middle aged and older adults. **Eight to 10 ounces of juice seems to be effective,** according to Dr. John D. Folts of the University of Wisconsin Medical School. His research has been funded by the Nutricia Research Foundation of the Netherlands and the Oscar Rennebohm Foundation of Madison, Wis., and more recently by **Welch's,** which makes grape juice

totally clear. Save your money and buy the real thing! All those "nutrients" and antioxidants won't make up for a fatty, salty diet that is low in fruits and vegetables.

A 16 year old who is anxious to "bulk-up" should avoid all those supplements and protein powders, creatine, taurine, and instead work-out with weights and eat my recommended diet. The slick advertisements found in sports magazines easily seduce teenagers as well as parents into believing the benefits promoted by these multivitamin, minerals, amino acids, protein drinks and powders, etc. Trainers supplement their income by suggesting that these kids need a high protein diet to build muscle because they are growing so rapidly and expending more energy than the average adolescent. The main beneficiaries of supplements sold in health food stores and gyms to teens are the pocket books of the purveyors of these pills and powders.

In the U.S., fresh fruit is usually available year round, but frozen and canned fruit are also nutritious. Although fruit loses some vitamins during the canning process, the loss is less than found in canned vegetables. This is because fruits are processed at lower temperatures, which destroys fewer nutrients. Try to avoid fruit canned in heavy syrup since it contains fewer vitamins and more sugar calories. Select water-packed canned fruit or canned fruit in unsweetened juice. Frozen strawberries, blueberries, cherries, and peaches are processed without cooking, and therefore there is little nutrient loss.

Dried fruits are an excellent source of vitamins, mineral, and fiber. Dried prunes, raisins, apricots, peaches and apples are available[50] in all markets. If possible, purchase the no-sulfite-added variety. Mild sulfite sensitivity or allergy may cause a slight tickling of the throat, while severe reactions can result in asthma or breathing difficulty. Check the health food stores for sulfite-

[50] Mariani Premium Mixed Fruit is a blend of dehydrated sliced apple, pitted prunes, apricots, freestone peaches, and Bartlett pears. Mariani Packing Co. Inc. 320 Jackson Street, San Jose, CA95112.

free dried fruit. If you're not sulfite sensitive, variety packs that contain sulfites[51] are available in most supermarkets.

Although the incidence of sulfite sensitivity is small in the general population, it can cause airway obstruction, cough, hives, and nasal congestion. The FDA banned the use of sulfites in fresh and raw fruit and vegetables in 1986. Commercial baby foods do not contain sulfites, but I do not recommend sulfite containing foods at any age, if it can be avoided. Certainly it should not be given to children with a history of hives or asthma. Sulfites are also commonly found in avocado dip, shrimp, shellfish, bacon and cold cuts. Federal law requires food manufacturers to list the sulfite content of any product containing more than ten parts per million. The FDA has a "generally recognized as safe" list (GRAS) that can give further information on sulfites.)

Prunes are a variety of dried plums. As with other dried fruit, the drying process concentrates the nutrients. First and foremost, prunes are a high-fiber food, containing ounce for ounce, more fiber than dried beans and most other fruits and vegetables. Over half this fiber is of the soluble blood cholesterol-lowering type. Prunes are also rich in beta carotene and are a good source of B vitamins, iron and potassium.

Like other dried fruit, raisins are a concentrated source of sticky-sugar calories, and supply 2 mgs of iron per 2/3 cup. That's 20% of the adult RDA for men and 13% of the adult RDA for women. That's as much iron, by weight, as cooked dried beans

[51] Sulfites are used widely by the food industry as a preservative and are found in processed potatoes, dried and packaged fruits and beverages, shrimp and seafood, beer and wine, avocado, guacamole, cider and vinegar, pickled vegetables, some albacore tuna, white grapes, maraschino cherries, fresh mushrooms, beet sugar, wet-milled corn and conditioned dough. Symptoms of sulfite allergy include mild tickling sensation of the throat to more severe reactions including tissue swelling, hives, cough, wheezing, asthma and rarely allergic shock. Researcher speculate that asthmatic sulfite reactions may be related to a deficiency of the enzyme sulfite oxidase, which is required to break down sulfite in the body. For more information: Asthma and Allergy Foundation of America, 1125 15th St., N.W. Suite 502, Washington, DC, 20005; Tel: 202-466-7643.

or ground beef. For the older child or adolescent raisins is a wholesome snack food. For the younger child, a diet of raisins along with excessive juice and crackers, often causes a skinny child with lots of tooth decay. So save this snack for the older child and don't forget to brush teeth afterwards.

To make a healthy low-fat trail mix, combine raisins with other dried fruit, puffed or shredded wheat cereal, popcorn, and sunflower seeds. Add spiced raisin into non-fat yogurt or add raisins and cinnamon to low fat or non-fat cottage cheese. Or pack plumped spicy raisins along with cinnamon into a pita bread pocket for a low-fat "Danish."

Real fruit juice is healthy, especially orange juice, but should be consumed in moderate amounts. Juices contain most of the fruit nutrients except for the very important fiber. Beverages labeled "juice" must be 100% juice. **Read the labels carefully!** "Juice blends," lemonade, fruit "punches," "drinks," and "juice cocktails," usually contain little juice, the rest being sugar water. Avoid Hi-C, Tang, Hawaiian Punch, GatorAid, Sunny Delight, V-8 Splash, Tropicana Twisters, Fruit soda and "Energy drinks". And don't get your child into the soda habit. **Soda is a poor choice because it destroys teeth, and its high phosphate content promotes calcium elimination from your body. There are 10 teaspoons of sugar in one can of Coke.** A growing body needs calcium for strong bone development. **Diet sodas** are a special hazard and should not be a part of your child's normal diet. Many parents mistakenly choose diet soda over regular soda because they believe sugar is a "poison." The important thing to remember about sugar is to consume only a little of it. When sugar becomes a major part of the diet, then it is harmful, as is any nutrient consumed in excess. The **long term effect** of artificial sweeteners has not been adequately studied, in my opinion, and therefore should be avoided by children and teenagers. Let's protect our children from nutritional experimentation!

A juice often overlooked is prune juice. This nutritious juice contains 3 mg of iron or 30% of the RDA for adult men, and

20% for women. A cup of prune juice contains 473 milligrams of potassium, about the same amount as eight pitted prunes. It contains a few more calories than orange juice, 182 calories per cup compared to 110 calories in a cup of orange juice. Don't purchase brands with added sugar. Be careful with any juice because it is a leading contributor to becoming overweight and obese.

When buying fruit, remember that fresh fruit tastes the best. If you are buying fruit to eat today, buy ripe. For tomorrow or the next day, look for fruit that needs just a little ripening. To hasten the ripening of pears and peaches, put them in a loosely closed paper bag at room temperature. I usually store them in the trunk of my car for a few days.

Fruit that continues to ripen in addition to peaches and pears: Apricots, bananas, cantaloupe, kiwi, nectarines, and plums.

Fruit to buy ripe and ready to eat: Apples, cherries, grapefruit, grapes, oranges, pineapple, strawberries, tangerines and watermelon.

THE OLDER CHILD'S DIET

▲ ▲ ▲

During elementary school years, children spend far more time away from home. School and outside activities consume a large part of each day. Peers, older children, baby-sitters and teachers influence your child's development. From these role models children pick up behaviors and habits - eating habits, as well as others. Sometimes parents begin to feel uneasy as they realize they have less control over what their children are doing and eating. With diet, as well as behavior in general, your chances of affecting the outcome will improve if you set a good example at home instead of resorting to criticism and threats.

One area that parents often question me about is school lunches. "What can I prepare for my child to take to school? It must be something convenient and transportable," they often ask. How can parents also make lunches nutritious and appealing? The latter is essential if you want to make sure your child won't trade the lunch you prepared for a bag of chips and cupcakes!

In my family we have dealt with the problem of school lunches for years. We have developed some good, nutritious recipes which have passed the test of time as well as the criteria for convenience. "Good food" need not be boring. Children need not feel deprived of life's goodies. Besides fresh fruits and fresh fruit juices, there are lots of nutritious low-salt, low-fat snacks easily prepared and commercially available. I will share them with you in the upcoming pages.

As a parent, you can become an activist whenever you see lots of junk food in a public or private school lunch program or at a PTA and after-school activities. Insisting that fresh fruit be offered alongside the snow cones, candy bars, chips, hot dogs, etc., won't make many inroads. These junk foods are too tempting for most children to resist, and the fruit will be left to rot. Your opponents will then remind you that your idealism is, "not practical." Don't accept such negativism. Armed with this book, you can explain why wholesome foods are practical, and when properly prepared and presented, are welcomed by children. Most parents realize their obligation to protect their children against the hazards of life. It is time to realize that junk foods are some of these hazards. In order to protect a child from falling into the habit of consuming large quantities of harmful foods, it is best not to have them available except for special occasions.

It is time I told you what I believe junk food is, if you haven't already guessed. To me junk food is one that contains an excess of calories from fat and sugar. In addition, salt is often a major ingredient, and fiber is usually absent or extremely low. **It is untrue that "junk foods" are void of nutrients. They often contain many nutrients, including protein, minerals, and vitamins. What makes them undesirable is the imbalance they bring to our diets.** Crackers, chips, hot dogs, salami, pepperoni pizza, ice cream, french fries, granola bars, Milky Ways, Lunchables, Hot Pockets[52] and Top Ramen are a few examples of disaster foods, loaded with salt and fats and depleted of fiber. If you

[52] Frozen sandwiches such as Hot Pockets ham and cheese are a 4-1/2 ounce, 340-calorie indulgence with 15 grams of fat and 840 milligrams of sodium.

don't believe that these foods have become the mainstay of our children's diet, look at a typical week's menu from an elementary or high school, public or private, in your community. I'm not suggesting that these foods never be consumed. They can be enjoyed as party or holiday foods. Daily consumption is what makes junk foods dangerous.

When I first began cooking for myself as a graduate student in Philadelphia during the 1950's, the supermarket visit was an adventure in gastro-chemistry. What were the food technologists coming out with today? I examined the shelves with the same glee I felt going to debut new cars.

Instant rice and instant mashed potatoes. One minute oatmeal and wheat cereal. Chocolate cake and bake mix in a jiffy. Instant chocolate pudding. All my favorites now at my fingertips! Frozen turkey pot pie, ice cream, and canned peaches for a high living dinner.

Now I'm talking as a traitor about these foods. They did carry me through hard times. The nutritional ravages against my body by my chosen diet was not visible, so who knew? What I didn't realize then is that it isn't significantly more time consuming or difficult to eat healthy foods. It takes only moments to wash a fresh ripe peach or peel an orange.

Like other physicians of my generation, we smoked cigarettes and over-consumed most of the foods I am now condemning. We were completely ignorant of the connection between diet and what we called degenerative diseases of adulthood, which we believed were inevitable. It wasn't until I completed my formal medical training that I learned about the **lipid hypothesis**[53] **and how inflammation can be triggered by a high fat diet**. <u>This gradually changed my approach to nutrition from a biochemical</u>

[53] Research has expanded our understanding of the atherosclerotic process. It has validated the Lipid Hypothesis and has discovered additional factors contributing to the development of atherosclerosis. A diet high in saturated fat is a major cause of clogged blood vessels and inflammation of our blood vessels often leads to heart attack and stroke. See Part II, The Chemical of Life, page 144 for more information on the Lipid Hypothesis.

concept to actual food choices. It is clear that with all the new nutritional information, our children have an opportunity to enjoy the rewards of improved health and vigor throughout adulthood. As parents, we have the obligation to provide the best we can for our children. One does not have to be wealthy to provide the best nutrition. In fact, healthy foods often cost less than many of the expensive processed meals passed off as food.

BREAKFAST

Many families face a time crunch getting to work or school in the morning. Children often try to capture that last moment of sleep before getting up for school, or teenagers may be more interested in hair or makeup, so there is seldom time for breakfast. It is estimated that 50-70 percent of students go to school without breakfast and that an adequate breakfast is consumed in no more than 20 percent of American households. Some youngsters have grown so accustomed to not eating breakfast that they don't feel hungry until midmorning.

So the question comes up–just how important is breakfast? My answer is an unequivocal **VERY**! Studies on school children show a strong link between a nutritious breakfast and improved school performance. Furthermore, the studies reveal that school performance is adversely affected by omitting breakfast. Children who skip breakfast seem to be more jumpy, have a harder time relating to peers and teachers, and have difficulty concentrating. The physiological reasons for these behavioral changes are poorly understood to date, but repeated observations have made them impossible to dismiss.

It's logical to assume that similar behavior and performance changes occur in adults who do not take the time to eat an adequate breakfast. For most people the time span between dinner and breakfast is anywhere from eleven to thirteen hours. Omitting breakfast adds another three hours to that fast. Fasting for this length of time puts a stress on the body and causes the formation of fatty acids which are released into the bloodstream. Free fatty acids contribute to the atherosclerotic process that damages and rapidly ages our blood vessels. Fasting also strains the gallbladder, which may lead an adolescent or adult to become more susceptible to a gallbladder attack. It is not my wish to deny the spiritual benefits of fasting to anyone whose religion recommends it for "cleansing the spirit", but there is no scientific evidence to recommend fasting from the nutritional point of view.

Breakfast on the run is one way of dealing with late starters, short of complete behavior modification. By that I mean a glass of 1% or non-fat milk, a banana and a whole wheat bagel with a wedge of low fat Laughing Cow Cheese smeared on it! Peel and eat the banana on the way to school. Add a hard boiled egg for more protein. Another alternative is a smoothie—4 oz. glass of real orange juice blended with a banana, strawberries or ripe pears, plus 3 oz. of 1% or non-fat milk.

Instant cooked cereal such as Oatmeal, Cream of Rice, Quick Cream of Wheat, Pillsbury Farina and Quinoa, may work if one has a little more time. Yes, they are very processed, and because these cereals are so highly processed, the fiber has been milled out, unlike regular oatmeal which contains an appreciable amount of fiber. Replace the fiber by adding fresh fruit, such as blueberries to the cereal. Remember what we discussed earlier. Until the food industry comes on board, compromise is a must to maintain parental sanity. So add hot water or milk and serve! The protein content of an average serving made with 4 oz. of non-fat milk is a respectable 8 grams. These cereals are low in fat and high in complex carbohydrates, with no sugar added.

Such cereals as Quaker 100% Natural, Heartland, and some Granola are extremely high in fat and sugar. These cereals boast "naturalness," but oils and sugars have been added—a not so natural occurrence. Since a high fat diet is more responsible for malnutrition in America than dietary deficiency, most high fat cereals should be avoided. **Read the labels on the boxes and select cereals with no more than 3 grams of fat per serving.**

Dry cereals have won a place in the traditional American breakfast. Some observers have stated the nutritional value of dry cereal is proportional to the amount of milk used with each serving. In many instances this is true. However, some of the dry cereals offer better nutrition than others. It is important to read labels on dry cereals since most overuse simple carbohydrates such as sucrose, corn syrup, fructose, HFCS, honey or molasses. Froot Loops, Cocoa Puffs, Sugar Pops, Cap'n Crunch and Honey Combs are but a few of the cereals to avoid. Of the dry cereals, Barbara's Shredded Wheat or high fiber Cranberry, Kashi Go Lean and Heart to Heart are cereals that rate favorably because most are low in fat and simple sugar and have some fiber.

Instant breakfast bars are really candy bars masquerading as food. Sports bars contain large amounts of sugar in the form of fructose, honey, molasses, corn syrup, dextrose, maltose, sorbitol, corn solids and lactose as discussed earlier. Most of these products are 40-70% simple carbohydrate when totaled. Not only do these sticky carbohydrates promote tooth decay, but they provide a high degree of calories without the natural nutrients of real food.[54] Many of these bars are low in fiber, compared with the usual amount of fiber accompanying equivalent calories found in real food. They will push your child closer to an early metabolic syndrome. Their sodium content is often excessive as well. Check nutrition labels for sugars, fat content and fiber. The Nutrition Facts and ingredients label may be more revealing than the hype on the wrapping. It's true that a child may be eager to eat these breakfast bars, while hot cereal causes a lengthy debate; but the result is instant poor dietary habit. The next time you're shopping, check the ingredients on the Pop Tart package. The first nine ingredients are sugars and then comes the trace of "dried apples." Even the low fat variety is an expensive jelly sandwich on toast.

[54] To learn more about carbohydrates, turn to Chapter on Carbohydrates for a quick refresher course.

As for pancake mixes, most contain too much salt and fat. It is estimated that three pancakes, about 4 inches in diameter with a patty of melted butter on each, provides 37 grams of fat and well over 1000 mg of sodium. Pancakes are a favorite for children and adolescents alike. Fortunately it is not hard to prepare a nutritious pancake. Select a low fat, low or reduced salt mix. Many new ones arrive on the shelves monthly. If the recipe calls for milk, use non-fat milk. Reduce the suggested oil by a third, and if directions call for an egg to be added, substitute two egg whites and discard the yolk. Use a non-stick ungreased frying pan or griddle.

To make good pancakes, the non-stick pan must be sufficiently heated. If it is not hot enough, the pancakes will be tough, since pancakes must be cooked rapidly; however, be careful to avoid making the pan hot enough to burn them. Test the temperature by dropping a few drops of water in the pan—it should sizzle immediately.

A breakfast favorite of mine is *palatschincken*, an Austrian crepe or pancake. It's easy to make. Prepare a low fat, low salt pancake mix but add more liquid to thin the mix. Pour about one tablespoon into a hot non-stick pan. Allow it to spread very thinly over an area about five inches in diameter. Turn it over and cook briefly. Remove the thin crepe from the pan and place on a dish. Put a tablespoon of your favorite fresh berries in the middle and roll it up as a blintz or tortilla. Sprinkle with a little powdered sugar. Try it on a relaxed Sunday morning. It's especially delicious when it's raining or snowing outside!

PIZZA

Pizza is probably the most popular main dish in American, so I won't suggest that you give it up. This gooey cheese and tomato sauce plus pepperoni topping fast food is the mainstay of many school lunch programs. It is promoted heavily as a high source of protein, vitamins, minerals and complex carbohydrates, but what is omitted is that one portion of pizza often contains over 1000 mg of sodium and loads of artery clogging fat. Although every pizza is different, depending on the pizza parlor's recipe, many pizzas provide over 25-30 grams or 50% of its calories from fat. If it's a double cheese pizza with pepperoni or ground beef, there's even more fat, nitrites, and salt. In general, pizza is also very low in fiber unless it is loaded with vegetable toppings. Defenders of the school pizza remind us of all that calcium and protein pizza provides. You draw your own conclusions. In the meantime, there are alternatives. Tasty lower fat and lower sodium pizza is available.

The next time you're at the pizza parlor ask for a pizza with less cheese and a vegetarian topping instead of sausage or pepperoni.

CHICKEN NUGGETS AND FISH STICKS

Another high fat, high sodium favorite is the chicken nuggets, now becoming a mainstay in the school lunch. Kids love these dishes and there is no need to give them up. What must be done is to prepare them using tasty low fat, low sodium recipes. For example, "breast tenders" can be **baked** instead of deep fried and they are delicious. Compare this with Louis Rich's greasy Turkey Nuggets. Mrs. Paul's Low Fat and Low Sodium fish sticks are a great improvement over regular fish sticks and is another example of how innovative cooking can change a poorly conceived food into a wholesome dish. Keep checking the Nutrition Facts label and be sure to read Part II of this book for more information on how to interpret the label.

MAKING YOUNG FISH FANS

One of our most nutritious foods, fish and seafood, are most often greeted with a "yuk!", unless it is fried "fish & chips," fried "Filet of

Fish" dipped in a high fat Tartar sauce or the heart deadly seafoods such as heavily creamed New England clam chowder, lobster bisque, fried crab cakes and fried shrimp. What is it about wholesomely prepared fish and shellfish that makes it so unappetizing to children and adolescents? My feeling is that it's because fish is not introduced early enough into a child's diet. In my private pediatric practice, I see many Asian children, first generation, who are introduced to fish soups before their first birthday. They seem to love fish. I have not seen an increase in food allergy in these children, but children with eczema probably should avoid fish until they are much older and not before consulting with their pediatrician, dermatologist, or allergist.

While many adults seem to be eating more fish recently, children need to be encouraged to sample foods such as broiled, grilled or baked salmon, bass, or shrimp and scallops saute' (using olive instead of butter) or kabobs.

Introduce fish soups to your children when they are young. "Tastes" are developed early. When I worked in Vietnam I noticed that children and adults ate fish soup for breakfast! My first reaction was, "How could they?" By the end of my first week of work at the Children's Hospital #1 in HoChiMinh City (Saigon), I was enjoying the traditional breakfasts of Pho (a chicken soup with rice noodles, shrimp or chicken) or fish soup.

COOKING TIP: Try the recipe for "FRIED" FILLET OF FISH

TREE NUTS AND SEEDS

Unsalted almonds and walnuts make nutritious snacks and should be a part of a prudent diet. They are high in protein and essential fatty acids. Almonds are a good source of omega-6 fats as found in vegetable oils. Walnuts on the other hand are rich in omega-3 fatty acids, the same type that comes from salmon and fatty fish. A 4-6 gram serving contain 95% of the daily value of omega-3 fatty acids. Unfortunately, too few children and teenagers eat nuts regularly. A small handful of almonds or walnuts can provide filling protein, fiber, unsaturated fats plus vitamins and minerals. They lower cholesterol levels and the anti-inflammatory power of omega-3 fatty acid may be cardio-protective. Other unsalted nuts include hazelnuts, Brazil nuts, pecans, pistachios, and cashews. But beware! Nuts are also small bundles of calories and avoid the salted versions.

For older children don't forget **seeds,** such as unsalted sunflower and pumpkin seeds.

The Food and Drug Administration (FDA) only allows food companies to say evidence "suggest but does not prove" that eating nuts reduces heart disease risk.

For those parents who don't want to cook or don't have time to cook there is always "take out." AVOID FAST FOOD TAKE OUT!!

In northern California there are many supermarkets besides Whole Foods that sell "take out" wholesome food choices. They are not inexpensive and unfortunately this eliminates or limits the choices for many low-income families.

IDEAS FOR SNACKS & LUNCHES AT HOME OR AFTER SCHOOL

These are suggestions when you run out of ideas

1. Grilled cheese sandwich using low-fat sliced Swiss or Jack cheese on toasted whole grain bread. Use a non-stick skillet

or microwave to melt the cheese. Low-fat and reduced fat cheese tastes better if it is melted.

2. Meat, brown rice and ketchup mix packed in Tupperware-like container for transportation. (see recipe page). Quinoa may be substituted for rice.

3. Baked apple plain, or with yogurt. (recipe page)

4. Meatloaf sandwich.

5. Tuna salad sandwich made with 50% less salt tuna and reduced or non-fat mayonnaise or low-fat yogurt. Make with a whole wheat slice of bread on one side and white bread on the other side.

6. Fresh fruit salad.

7. Bowl of low sodium chili, vegetarian or with very lean meat (refer to recipe included earlier.)

8. Chicken sandwich using low salt ketchup as a spread, or reduced-fat mayonnaise. Corn-on-the-cob. When not in season, a bowl of washed frozen corn kernels mixed with green peas. (Look for no added sugar brands). A zip-lock type bag makes this mixture transportable.

9. Boca Burger or Veggie Burger (vegetarian "hamburger" found in most health food stores-frozen section) grilled, and served on a toasted bun with low sodium ketchup, slice of butter lettuce and slice of **ripe** tomato. Use sliced cherry tomatoes when vine ripened tomatoes are not available.

10. Extra lean roast beef sandwich with favorite whole grain roll. Use mustard or ketchup as a spread. Serve with a banana or slice of melon. Have a side dish of small boiled potatoes, broccoli florets, and sliced steamed carrots.

11. Hamburger made with **extra** lean ground beef. Add some rice or quinoa and chicken broth to the meat mixture to keep it moist and enhance its flavor. For variety try mixing in a little mustard or bar-BQ sauce. Serve with low salt brand of chicken with rice noodle soup. Add an apple or seasonal fruit.

12. Meat loaf sandwich (use included recipe for low fat meat loaf) Raw carrots and cherry tomatoes. Mixed dehydrated fruit (Mariani Premium Mixed Fruit is a blend of dehydrated sliced apple, pitted prunes, apricots, freestone peaches, and Bartlett pears. Mariani Packing Co. Inc. 320 Jackson Street, San Jose, CA 95112)

13. Cup of pea soup using one of the many low-sodium, low-fat brands. Baked skinless drumettes of chicken, sprinkled with sweet paprika over rice. Slice of cantaloupe or cubes in a bowl with blueberries when in season.

14. Boiled, steamed or microwaved corn on the cob, without any salt, but a little "I Can't Believe It's Not Butter," if desired. Broiled skinless chicken breast, plain or sliced thin on a bun with fresh salsa as a topping. Fresh orange, peeled.

15. Small bowl of macaroni with grated non-fat cheese, such as Kraft shredded reduced-fat mozzarella, sprinkled over it and microwaved until the cheese melts. Low sodium vegetable soup. A fruit smoothie (limit to only once a week).

16. Ravioli (Soy Boy) Plain, Ravioli Rosa, Ravioli Verde (Northern Soy, Inc. 545 West Ave., Rochester, New York 14611, 1-716-235-8970.) A great snack as well as a lunch! Serve with a small salad. Dried mixed fruit, such as raisins, apple, pear, and apricot.

17. Nachos (a low fat recipe is included) Bowl of low fat, low sodium beans. (Don't forget the **Beano** - 2-3 drops with the first bite!) Strawberry-banana smoothie.

18. Fresh toasted whole wheat bagel with Hummus or low-fat whipped cream cheese. One tablespoon of cooked bay shrimp stirred into a cup of minestrone soup (Low-sodium brand). Raw celery and raw carrots. Edamame-cooked soy beans (pronounced "eh-dah-MAH-may) are fun to eat and easy to serve. Add a hard boiled egg.

19. Bowl of medium sized shrimp and salsa (recipe included). Baked potato with lowfat sour cream and chives. (**Naturally Yours Fat Free Sour Cream*** is especially delicious and has 67% less calories than regular sour cream.) Use salsa as topping for potato as well, if desired. Hungarian cucumber salad. (recipe included)

*Naturally Yours Fat Free Sour Cream is distributed by M STAR INC. 5956 Sherry Lane, Dallas, TX 75225. Contains 30 calories/serving; 25 mg sodium; 2 grams protein and only 2 grams of sugar.

20. Leftover wholewheat spaghetti or macaroni with low sodium, low fat tomato meat sauce. Serve heated or cold. Transportable in a "Tupperware-like" container. Fresh apple. 1% milk. Avoid chocolate milk because it contains 14 grams (about 3-1/2 teaspoons) of added sugar!

21. Turkey sandwich made with unprocessed real turkey.[55] (avoid the highly processed high sodium turkey rolls). Use low-fat mayonnaise or cranberry sauce as a spread. Mashed potato, baked yam or sweet potato.

22. Pita bread (pocket bread) stuffed with shredded lettuce, cooked ground lean hamburger meat or cooked ground turkey, and low fat salad dressing on top.

23. Beef or turkey tacos with shredded lettuce, tomato, shredded non-fat or low-fat cheese. Glass of non-fat or 1% milk. Whole

[55] Avoid the salted turkey roll or pre-wrapped processed chicken or turkey slices.

wheat fig bars (Pride O the Farm Fat Free) or a no sugar added brand.[56]

24. Cold leftover broiled salmon sandwich served with low fat salad dressing as a spread, lettuce and slice of ripe tomato. A salmon salad with medley of vegetables is another variation.

25. Omelet made with two egg whites and one yolk. Cubed vegetable sauté, shredded mozzarella cheese, and lean low-sodium ham, diced for the inside. Served with salsa over the top when cooked. Serve with a fresh whole wheat toasted bagel and very small boiled new potatoes.

26. Egg salad sandwich (see included recipe). Unsalted or low sodium whole wheat pretzels.

27. Chili dog (Nitrite free hot dog[57] on a toasted bun with non-fat chili beans spooned over it. Non-fat corn chips. Or Aidells Chicken & Apple: one link contains 180 calories; 12 grams protein; 2 grams sugar; 85 mg cholesterol; 0 trans fats; 640 mg sodium, nitrite free, saturated fat 3.5 grams. Calories from fat 110.)

28. Waffles made with low-fat pancake mix or Buckwheat Pancakes using above recipe. (Goldrush[58], San Francisco Style, Sour Dough reduced fat Pancake & Waffle Mix. Recipe on box.)

29. Gazpacho-especially on those warm days. Enchilada or taco. No sour cream on top.

30. Banana bread, corn bread or potato latkes with apple sauce.

---

[56] The sugars number on the label includes naturally occurring sugars in fruit as well as added sugar. That's frustrating if you want to know how much came from the fig in the Newtons.

[57] They usually employ celery powder or celery juice which is high in nitrates! So beware of this deception. Make hot dogs a very rare treat.

[58] Goldrush Sour Dough Pancake & Waffle Mix. Cal-Gar 383 Beach Road, Burlingame, CA 94010.

31. Wanda's spaghetti pie. (recipe section)

32. Sliced kiwi, dry cereal (Shredded Wheat, Kashi Heart to Heart) and non-fat or 1% milk.

33. Turkey hamburger (see included recipe) Fresh orange slices or mandarin wedges.

34. Teriyaki fish sandwich (see included recipe). **Small** bag of low-fat, low sodium, corn or potato chips. Grapes or seasonal melon.

35. Bay Shrimp tacos with shredded lettuce, chopped onion and very ripe tomato, cilantro plus tomatillo sauce topping. Craisins, figs and other dried fruit.

36. Low-fat bean burrito (see included recipe), slice of watermelon if in season or Carol's banana shake (recipe included)

37. Salmon sandwich on rye or whole wheat bread. (Canned salmon mixed with low-fat mayo and chopped scallions plus sliced cherry tomatoes with butter lettuce on top.)

38. Spread one teaspoon of low-fat herbal whipped cream cheese on a whole wheat tortilla. Place 1-2 slices of unsalted, sliced real roasted turkey on it and roll it up. This makes a great breakfast or snack.

39. Substitute 100% orange juice (limit OJ only once or twice a week) for a Capri Sun drink. Avoid beverages that say, "drink" or "punch" "lemonade," because most have little more nutrition than colored sugar water.

40. Don't forget the ten super-foods: Sweet potatoes, whole grain bread, broccoli, strawberries, beans, cantaloupe, spinach and kale, oranges, oatmeal, fat-free (skim) or 1% fat milk.

THE FOODS CHILDREN NEED, PART 2

▲ ▲ ▲

FISH AND SHELLFISH

Tuna, pollack, cod, salmon, and flounder account for at least three-quarters of all the fish Americans eat. Other varieties such as bass, catfish, shark, trout, monkfish, orange roughy, swordfish, and Mahi-mahi are growing in popularity. Although some fish are slightly high in fat, most fish are an excellent source of low cholesterol, low saturated fat, and high protein, and should be consumed more often by children, adolescents and adults. Some children enjoy fish from an early age while others seem to acquire a taste for fish a little later. This may be cultural, since most of my Asian and Hispanic patients seen to enjoy fish and shellfish by one year of age.

Unfortunately, fish sticks, "Fillet O Fish," fish ' n chips, and other types of fried fish appeal to children too. Fish sticks are coated with crumbs or batter, fried and frozen. Because they are easy to reheat in the microwave, they appear to be a simple and nutritious answer to preparing fish. Although fish sticks and these fried fish products are an excellent source of protein they are made with pollock, an inexpensive fish very low in omega-3 fat [59]and they are coated with as much as 13 grams of fat or about 45% calories from fat. There's also a lot of added sodium-more than 900 mg per serving in some brands. Add salty ketchup, tartar sauce or cocktail sauce and you're already exceeding the daily total Nutritional Guidelines recommendation for salt. If you do buy fish sticks, look for brands that say baked low-fat and low-sodium. They should contain four grams of fat per serving or less and half the salt found in regular fish sticks. For example, Mrs. Paul's Low Fat Fish Sticks contains 4 grams of fat and 450 mg of salt per five-stick serving. This is a reasonable compromise if you're looking for something easy to prepare after an exhausting day. Check the Nutrition Facts label. I've included several fish recipes that most children love, such as Red Snapper Veracruzana, Fish stew, and "Shake ' N Bake" preparations of shrimp, whitefish, and scallops. My mock crab dipped in cocktail sauce recipe is another favorite of older children, teenagers, and young adults. Since crab is not a "kosher" food and therefore not eaten by many observant Jews, many Jewish cook books contain excellent tasty recipes for making imitation crab snacks or meals.

Fish provides more than relatively low-fat protein. It is high in DHA docosahexaenoic acid, which is the fatty acid (a component of fat) that is needed for optimal brain growth and eye development. (Refer to the earlier chapter on breastfeeding and breast milk.). EPA (eicosapentaenoic acid), another fatty acid found in fish lowers blood cholesterol and protects arterial walls against the harmful effect of LDL cholesterol. These compounds are referred to as omega-3 fatty acids (These "fats"

[59] Omega-3-fatty acids is another name for linolenic fatty acids, found in plants and cold-water fish. Omega-6 and Omega 3-fatty acids are special essential fats (found in fish, nuts, flaxseed and certain vegetable oils). See the next page and the section on fats, Part II: pages 141-142. Also see alpha-linolenic acid (ALA); docosahexanoic acid (DHA); and Eicosapentenoic acid (EPA).

are referred to as "fish oils.") and are also found in shellfish. Another or second variety of omega-3 fatty acid, *alpha-linolenic acid* is found in plant foods and is especially high in oils such as canola oil. This essential fatty acid (a fat that the body can't manufacture) is needed for the growth and maintenance of our cells, tissues, and entire body. Inside the body, a small amount of *alpha-linolenic acid* is converted to EPA and DHA. As described in Part I of this book under the Science of Nutrition, there is another essential fatty acid. It is called *linoleic acid.* Foods high in linoleic acid are vegetable oils such as corn, safflower, soybean and sunflower seed oils. Most of us eat ten times as much linoleic acid as alpha-linolenic acid. It is believed that the ratio should be closer to 1: 1. When linoleic acid dominates too heavily over the omega-3s (alpha-linolenic acid, DHA, and EPA) we may be more prone to illness that cause inflamed muscles and joints, increased menstrual cramps, heart arrhythmias (irregular heart beats), and even post-partum depression. **A 3 ounce serving of baked salmon provides almost 2 grams of EPA plus DHA. That is 10 times the calculated current intake found in the average American diet.** If you don't like fish, substitute your polyunsaturated salad oil, (corn, safflower, or soybean oil) with a plant omega-3 oil such as canola oil. Remember, though, it is important to keep total fat low, and if you follow my diet suggestions you will automatically consume sufficient essential fatty acids or fats.

As much as I believe fish is an important part of the diet, pregnant women should avoid fatty fish such as sablefish, mackerel, bluefish, and stripped bass because they contain pesticides, mercury, and cancer-causing PCB's. Eat swordfish, or fresh tuna steaks no more than once a week due to the possibility of an elevated mercury content. A 1994 study of San Francisco Bay waters found unsafe methyl mercury levels in some fish caught in those waters, prompting warning that consumption of these fish be severely restricted. Pregnant women can avoid excess mercury by limiting consumption of canned tuna to seven ounces a week. Any freshwater fish caught in inland lakes, especially the Great Lakes are more likely to be contaminated with PCB's and dioxin and should be completely avoided especially during pregnancy. PCB's also have been shown to contribute to learning problems in children.

FISH OIL-omega -3 fatty acids have recently been promoted to reduce inflammation (see Inflammation Hypothesis) and thus protect the heart from a "sudden" heart attack and cellular aging. The current recommendation is to consume two fish meals a week, preferably dark fleshed fish that is high in omega -3 fatty acids (Arctic Char, Mackerel, and Herring).

COOKING TIP: Try the recipe for "FRIED" FILLET OF FISH

MEATS AND POULTRY

Americans love meat! Meat and poultry are the central focus of most of our meals. Meat is high in saturated fat and cholesterol, especially beef, pork, and lamb. In recent years consumers have been made aware that a diet high in meat is associated with colon and prostate cancer and increases the risk of an early heart attack, the number one cause of death for American men and women. Does that mean you should not eat meat?

Children, adolescents, and adults can nutritionally benefit from a small amount of meat in their daily diet. The emphasis should be on small. For a teenager or adult, no more than 3-1/2 oz serving per day. That portion amounts to the size of a deck of cards. Meats and poultry are exceptionally rich in iron, zinc, and vitamins B-6 and B-12. These nutrients are difficult to obtain in a meatless diet. The choice of meat or poultry should be low in fat - less than 10 grams of fat per 3-1/2 oz serving. I will list these foods below with their approximate fat content, so you will be able to make a nutritionally intelligent choice when selecting meats for your family meal, at home, your favorite fast food take-out, or restaurant.

COMPARING BEEF CUTS

Ground Beef: 3-1/2 ounces cooked

	Calories	Fat grams	Saturated fat grams	Cholesterol(mg)
Regular ground beef:	**289**	**21**	**8**	**90**
Lean ground beef:	**272**	**18**	**7**	**87**
Extra lean ground beef	**256**	**16**	**6**	**84**

As you can see by the above table, cholesterol levels do not change very much between regular beef and extra lean ground beef. It is the fat content that does change, and fat is more atherogenic (more damaging to the blood vessels) than cholesterol. Therefore, concentrate on decreasing the total fat content of your food choices. When broiling or grilling hamburger, it is important to thoroughly cook the meat until there is no "pink meat," and the juices should be brown. This will ensure that any harmful contaminating bacteria have been killed.

Beef Cuts: 3-1/2 ounces completely trimmed of external fat.

	Calories	Fat grams	Saturated fat grams	Cholesterol (mg)
Eye of round, choice	**175**	**6**	**2**	**69**
Tip round, choice	**180**	**6**	**2**	**81**
Top round, choice	**207**	**6**	**2**	**90**
Sirloin, choice	**200**	**8**	**3**	**89**
Brisket	**218**	**10**	**4**	**93**
T-Bone steak, choice	**214**	**10**	**4**	**80**
Porterhouse steak, choice	**218**	**11**	**4**	**80**
Tenderloin[60], choice	**212**	**10**	**4**	**84**

60 Cuts of beef that end with the word, "loin,"as in tenderloin, is one of the leaner cuts.

Ribs, whole, choice	**237**	**14**	**6**	**77**
Short ribs, choice	**298**	**18**	**8**	**93**

When selecting beef, look for cuts that have little marbling and external fat. Ask the butcher to trim away all visible fat. At home, trim fat before cooking. This external fat is the biggest source of fat in beef. This fat trimming has no effect on tenderness, flavor or juiciness of the meat.

In low fat cooking, beef can be served as a "side dish" rather than the main part of the meal. The serving for an adolescent or young adult may be about 3-1/2 ounces or the size of a deck of cards. For the younger child, the serving should be less.

LAMB

Lamb is relatively high in fat. The best way to estimate the fat content is the cut. The information below assumes that all cuts have been trimmed of external fat.

Ground lamb is very high in fat. If you want to lower the content of fat in ground lamb, have the butcher trim lamb shoulder and grind it. This will reduce in half the fat content from approximately 20 grams of fat per 3-1/2 ounces to 11 grams.

COMPARING LAMB CUTS

3-1/2 ounces cooked

	Calories	Fat (grams)	Saturated fat (grams)	Cholesterol(mg)
Shank	**180**	**7**	**2**	**87**
Leg	**191**	**8**	**3**	**89**
Loin	**202**	**10**	**4**	**87**
Shoulder	**204**	**11**	**4**	**87**

Blade	209	12	4	87
Rib	232	13	5	88

PORK

"The other white meat"

Pork is not as lean as skinless chicken breast, turkey breast, or fish. However, if you eat small portions and pay attention to trimming away all visible fat, and stay with lean cuts, pork provides many important nutrients. Pork is an excellent source of thiamine, zinc, iron, and high quality protein. Bacon, sausage, spareribs, and hot dogs are extremely high in fat, salt and nitrites. Ham is also high in salt and nitrites. These nitrites combine with protein during cooking and produce *nitrosamins,* which are linked to stomach cancer. These foods should be reserved for very special occasions and not be daily fare for your children or yourself.

COMPARING PORK CUTS

3-1/2 ounces trimmed and cooked

	Calories	Fat (grams)	Saturated Fat (grams)	Cholesterol (mg)
Bacon[61]	576	49	17	85
Spareribs	395	30	11	121
Blade loin	247	15	5	93
Country style	234	14	5	86
Loin	200	9	3	79
Tenderloin	164	5	2	79
Ham, canned[62]	155	5	2	30

[61] **Three slices equals an ounce of cooked bacon and it contains 110 calories, and 9 grams of fat which is 74% of calories from fat**

[62] Three and one half ounces of bacon contains a whopping 1000 mg of sodium!

SAUSAGES

Sausages are very high in fats, salts and stomach cancer producing nitrites and nitrates.

Eat them sparingly and try to convince your misguided PTA to stop using these foods to raise money.

Use sausages as a flavoring for foods, rather than the main course.

Gourmet sausages are appearing at many markets. Labels that brag "95% fat free" may actually contain many fat grams along with nitrites and a high sodium content. Before buying these tempting delicacies, read the Nutrition Facts plus Ingredients to get beyond the promotional hype. If you choose to eat them occasionally, be sure to decrease that day's fat allowance by preparing meals with high fiber, low fat, low sodium foods.

COMPARING SAUSAGES

3-1/2 ounces

	Calories	Fat	Sodium
Pepperoni, beef & pork	**500**	**45**	**2000**
Pork sausage, fresh, cooked	**370**	**30**	**1300**
Chorizo, beef & pork	**450**	**38**	**1200**
Kielbasa	**310**	**27**	**1000**
Liverwurst, pork	**325**	**29**	**850**
Hot dogs (2), beef & pork	**320**	**29**	**1100**
Hot dogs (2), chicken	**255**	**19**	**1350**
Salami, beef & pork	**250**	**20**	**1000**
Bologna, pork	**245**	**20**	**1100**
Bologna, turkey	**200**	**15**	**675**

Canned ham, Canadian bacon, and cured ham all contain about 1000 mg of sodium.

CHICKEN

Not all the chicken we eat is low in fat. Eating chicken **with the skin** will more than double the amount of fat. Chicken skin has 80% of its calories from fat, and over 20% is from saturated fat. Dark meat contains more fat than white meat and is slightly higher in cholesterol as well. Most children love chicken, and it is an extremely versatile meat. There are recipe books devoted entirely to chicken. Consult them and don't be afraid to alter the recipes by decreasing or eliminating any added cream, butter, margarine or oil.

A busy parent can buy skinless chicken breast fillets, fresh or frozen. Instant "gourmet" meals, such as Kim's Chicken, as well as low-fat nuggets can be prepared with minimal effort.

A chicken favorite among children is McDonald's Chicken McNuggets[63]. These Nuggets are loaded with 15 grams of fat, with 50% of calories from fat! Conscientious parents who want to give their child "the best of the worst" mistakenly choose McNuggets or the fried fish. A lower fat choice is a hamburger without cheese and a carton of milk instead of the soda. If you must buy the fries, which are loaded with the artery damaging fats, settle for a small order to share.

Chicken liver is another favorite that should be avoided. Although it is relatively low in fat, 3-1/2 ounces contains 630mg of cholesterol, double the maximum daily amount of cholesterol recommended for adults. And that's not all. The liver is an organ that concentrates all toxins and therefore may contain higher levels of pesticides. Pesticides often contaminate the grains fed to the chickens or seeds eaten by "organic" or free range chickens, since DDT and other pesticides remain in the soil for years.

[63] If you buy the batter-dipped chicken breast and want to turn it into a healthier meal, remove all the skin. Taking off the skin removes about 8 grams of fat from a chicken breast. A deep fried chicken thigh has 23 grams of artery clogging fat. Skip the onion rings (19grams of fat) and the coleslaw (11 grams fat in a _ cup serving).

Eating less red meat does not mean your child should eat more chicken. The most important recommendation for healthy eating is to make vegetables, fruits and grain products the largest and most appetizing part of your family's diet.

COMPARING CHICKEN PARTS

3-1/2 ounces cooked

PART	Calories	Fat (gms)	Saturated fat (gms)	Cholesterol (mg)
Breast, with skin	**197**	**8**	**2**	**84**
Breast, without skin	**165**	**4**	**1**	**85**
Drumstick, with skin	**253**	**16**	**4**	**91**
Drumstick, without skin	**172**	**6**	**1**	**93**
Wing, with skin	**290**	**20**	**5**	**84**
Wing, without skin	**203**	**8**	**2**	**85**

Like beef, there is little difference between cuts and the cholesterol content of chicken. It is the high fat content of skin on the chicken versus skinned chicken that will make the major difference. Of course, fried chicken should be avoided, and if a recipe calls for sour cream, **use a non-fat sour cream or non-fat yogurt.**

TURKEY

Turkey breast is the leanest of all meats with 7% of calories from fat. Even turkey breast with skin has only 18% of calories from fat. Almost all of the fat in turkey is found in the skin. Dark turkey meat is higher in fat, but is relatively lean if eaten without the skin. Roaster and hen turkeys are good choices for broiling, roasting or grilling, as they are the most tender. Hens have a larger proportion of white to dark meat. Tom turkeys are larger and older than roasters or hens, and have a reputation for being tastier. Ground turkey is an excellent substitute for ground beef, but it usually needs more seasoning and moisture. Try fresh herbs to add both moisture and flavor. Egg white or tomato juice also enhances flavor and adds moisture to ground turkey. Packaged ground turkey often contains dark meat and may contain more fat, as much as 55% calories from fat. Be sure to check the Nutritional Guidelines on the label.

Avoid turkey rolls, and those turkey slices in "convenient" little bags. Instead choose sliced fresh turkey from your deli. "Lunchables" are to be avoided since they are loaded with salt, nitrites, and are high in fat. There are healthier convenience foods available for your children.

COMPARING TURKEY PARTS

3-1/2 ounces cooked

	Calories	Fats (gms)	Saturated Fat (gms)	Cholesterol (mg)
Breast, without skin	**135**	**1**	**<1**	**83**
Breast, with skin	**153**	**3**	**1**	**90**
Dark meat without skin	**162**	**4**	**1**	**112**
Dark meat with skin	**182**	**7**	**2**	**117**
Leg with skin	**170**	**5**	**2**	**70**
Wing with skin	**207**	**10**	**3**	**115**

COOKING TIP: Try the recipes for LOW-FAT TURKEY GRAVY and TURKEY MEATBALLS

THE ADOLESCENT'S DIET[64]

▲ ▲ ▲

Adolescence may be defined as the teenage years between 12 and 20, but physical maturation and changes in nutrient requirements actually begin at younger ages and extend into young adulthood. The spurt of growth during adolescence is second only to the rate of growth during infancy, but less predictable. Every parent knows how important good nutrition is for their adolescent son or daughter and naturally turns to authorities such as physicians, dietitians, or "trainers," for guidance. Here

[64] The subjects of obesity and eating disorders such as anorexia nervosa and bulimia are extremely important since both often begin before the onset of puberty. However it is beyond the scope of this book to discuss adequately these important problems. Rather I would refer you to your physician to direct you to one of the many excellent up to date books available. For older adolescents, a useful formula for calculating ideal body weight based on barefoot height is:

Males: 5 feet = 106 lbs. + 6 lbs. Per additional inch.

Females 5 feet = 100 lbs. + 5 lbs. Per additional inch.

is where more confusion begins since nutrient allowances, or Recommended Daily Allowances for adolescents (RDA's) are only estimates or "educated guesses.[65]" Nutritionists took data on young children and adults, and applied it to adolescents without actually measuring their needs. The unusually tall teenager and the early maturer or late maturer will vary considerably in their needs. Their nutritional requirements (RDA's), therefore, should be looked upon more as "guidelines" and not embraced dogmatically. For example, a 14 year old boy may require 600 to 1200 milligrams of calcium a day, depending on absorption rates of 50% or 25%. The RDA of 1200mg of calcium per day, for example, is thus designed to meet the needs of the adolescent who is growing at the fastest rate. Levels less than that may be quite adequate for many teenagers. This explains the absence of problems in areas of the world where the daily intake is a minimal 200 to 300 mg of calcium per day.

Teenagers gain 50% of their bone mass during their pubertal growth spurt, and 90% of total body calcium is found in the skeleton (bones). Because most of a girl's bone mass in the spine and upper femur (thigh bone) is reached at age 16 years, anything that interferes with mineralization of bone during these critical growth years can have long-term consequences. This is the best age to prevent osteoporosis and future broken hips, especially since there are no good treatments for osteoporosis at the present time. It is between ages nine and twenty four that most children store calcium in their bones. These are the years when many adolescent girls favor diet drinks and consume little calcium rich dairy products. Osteoporosis is best prevented by maximizing calcium intake during these years. Encourage your teenager to drink non-fat milk or juice fortified with calcium to

---

[65] 15-18 year old girls is 44 grams while the average consumption is estimated to be 63 grams. The recommended dietary allowance of protein for 15-to-18-year-old boys is 59 grams, but studies have shown that it is not unusual for intakes to be well over 100 grams of protein a day.

get the needed amount of calcium. A vitamin D fortified calcium supplement may be needed if your child has an aversion to dairy products.

A high protein diet stresses the kidneys and causes calcium to be removed from the body. Even the leading nutritional experts of the World Health Organization recommend progressively decreasing levels of protein. It is no wonder that nutritional deficiency of protein, simple carbohydrate or fat is extremely rare among American teenagers. At highest risk for protein and calcium deficiency are teenagers on extreme weight loss diets, teens from poor families, and those who eat no animal products.

Many nutritionists, in their preoccupation with deficiency states, continue to proclaim in the lay and medical literature that fast foods or junk foods allow the vast majority of adolescents to maintain an adequate nutritional status, despite their erratic eating patterns. These nutritionists state that despite the pattern of skipped meals, or choosing pie or fried chicken over lower fat, high complex carbohydrate choices, teenagers will receive the necessary amounts of vitamins[66] and minerals because of the sheer quantity of food they consume. I hope by now, the reader will appreciate the absurdity of such notions. These apologists for the food industry claim that the links between salt and hypertension, high fat and cardiovascular disease, gallbladder disease, and some cancers are not conclusive. As an aside, the tobacco industry continues to make similar assertions. There are

---

66 Analysis of information from the Bogalusa Heart Study, as reported by Zive and colleagues in the Journal of Adolescent Health, 1996, pages 39-47, revealed that adolescents are most likely to be deficient in vitamins A, B-6, E, D, C, and folic acid. Mineral deficiencies were most common for iron, zinc, calcium, and magnesium. Adolescent girls were more likely than adolescent boys to have dietary deficiencies, due primarily to their decreased overall food consumption. Adolescents who are restricting their food intake to lose weight are at increased risk for vitamin and mineral deficiencies and might benefit from supplementation. This all may be true, but the over-consumption of artery clogging fats, sodium, and highly refined, low fiber foods must be revealed as the chief culprits of modern day malnutrition.

nutritionists who will tell you to consume all the salt you want, and this advice gets promoted on TV programs such as 20/20. They would have you believe that the major nutritional issues confronting teenagers relate to calcium, iron, and protein or vitamin A and C deficiency. This is a typical half truth. **No wonder parents are totally confused over what constitutes a nutritious diet. Experts, often aligned with the food industry, must share the responsibility for this confusion. Truth is the first victim when huge profits are at stake.**

Because of commercial hype and promotion, many adolescents incorrectly believe that the more protein in their diet the better.[67] But excess protein is not converted to muscle, it's converted into fat! As pointed out earlier most teenagers need **less** than 60 grams of protein a day (unless pregnant[68]or breastfeeding). While adolescent boys often overdose on protein, I'm concerned about those teenage girls who go in the other direction, under-consuming nutrients, while surviving on no-cal soda, chips, and candy or, "sports bars.

Fad diets seem to work–that is, weight is lost. The reason I'm taking time here is because so many teenage athletes are being sold by their coaches many of the bogus concepts detailed in "nutrition" books. Nutritional advice based on the "diet du jour" should be dismissed as yet another untested theory. Most are not sustainable for life, and the fad diet will soon fade into history. Unfortunately, it will probably be replaced by another one

---

[67] Pregnant teenagers have special nutritional needs because there are at least two growing bodies, the adolescent and the fetus. Protein requirements are increased by 10-15 grams per day, bringing the daily recommended protein intake to 60 grams per day. Most women in the United States, including those who might be at risk due to age or socioeconomic status, easily meet this level.

[68] Adolescent girls require approximately 0.36 grams of dietary protein daily per pound of body weight. Boys require about 0.45 grams of protein daily per pound of body weight. Most teens in this country meet or exceed this level, including teens on vegetarian diets.

filled with exaggerations based on half-truths, pseudo-science, and convincing anecdotes.

Another myth is that beef is the best protein. It certainly is an excellent source of iron, but fish, egg white, breast of chicken, and turkey are equally good sources and considerably lower in fat and cholesterol. Also plant protein from brown rice, quinoa, wheat, beans and corn are excellent sources of very low fat proteins. Non-fat milk, although often thought of as a "calcium food" is extremely rich in non-fat protein, although low in iron.

It is sometimes argued that teenage athletes need extra protein or a higher amount of a specific amino acid, such as "glutamine," and vitamins. [69]We've all seen the picture of the athlete sitting down to a big steak dinner during training. "Pure muscle building protein," in the form of supplements or meats does not increase strength or help build muscles. Muscle size and strength are developed by muscular work, not by eating meat or magical protein drinks. Extra complex carbohydrates, such as whole grain bread, brown rice, potato, whole grain cereals, pasta, vegetables, and fruit, are desirable to provide the extra energy for the muscular work and growth that go into muscle building. It is also rare for any healthy athlete to need salt tablets as a supplement to compensate for salt lost in perspiration. "Enzymes," DHEA (sold in many gyms alongside "High Performance" Ultra-whatever bars as a supplement) and "natural" multivitamin mixes promoted by coaches and trainers to the psychologically vulnerable teenager, and their parents, have as much nutritional value as a placebo. **"Power bars" are no substitute for real food.** The teenager may feel and say, "I took the protein vitamin drink and

[69] Supplements are part of a multi-billion dollar business. So when you're asked to swallow, in addition to wholesome fruits and vegetables, some anti-cancer or fitness "drink," remind the promoter what you've learned. So far there is no individual chemical, phytochemical, vitamin, mineral or amino acid, despite the endless parade of headlines and promotions, that has been proven to improve upon your performance, that adds to or is a substitute for a good diet and exercise. These specialty foods, pills or drinks are expensive "hope"-enriched potions.

immediately felt that power surge." But vitamins and minerals do not work that way. What they are reporting is the powerful placebo effect of suggestion. (or perhaps it contains lots of caffeine!).Wishful or magical thinking is powerful and often clouds the intellect. Trainers and gyms often supplement their incomes with the concoctions they sell. Such conflict of interest may get in the way of their usual good judgment. They often give you what I call a "nutrition-biochemistry babble" sales pitch, which sounds very convincing to anyone with a casual understanding of clinical nutrition.

Which brings me to another pseudo science fad: Ginkgo biloba, ginseng, guarana, chromium picolinate, vitamin B12, coenzyme Q10, and especially creatine. There is little or no scientific evidence to support the claims for most of these substances. The only pill or drink that will boost your energy is one containing a stimulant, such as caffeine, and the effects of these stimulants wear off within hours.

Ginkgo biloba has been used for centuries in Chinese medicine and its effect on thinking , mood, alertness, and memory have been subject to many studies, but many of these studies have been of poor quality. This is not the way to improve your memory.

Ginseng is a relatively safe herb. It is said to reduce fatigue and enhance stamina and endurance. Most research concludes it does not improve oxygen use or aerobic performance, or influence how quickly you bounce back after exercising.

Guarana is an herb that induces a feeling of energy because it is a natural source of caffeine.

Chromium picolinate is a trace mineral widely marketed to build muscle, burn fat, and increase energy and athletic performance. None of these claims are supported by research. Too bad it does not work that way.

DHEA is marketed as a "fountain of youth," and prevents cancer, heart disease, and infectious disease, among other things. Doesn't it make you want to run out and get some?

Unfortunately, the truth is that DHEA has no proven benefits and some potentially serious health risks, such as lowering levels of healthy HDL cholesterol, acne and facial hair in women.

Creatine is another supplement that many of my teenage patients say they take on the advice of their "trainer" to build muscle mass and improve athletic performance. While no adverse effects of taking creatine in doses of 2-3 grams per day as recommended on the bottle, there are very few studies of sufficient size and duration to allow confidence about the lack of adverse effects.

It is helpful to educate the athlete that the muscle and strength they are working so hard to gain is being broken down and used as an expendable fuel source. Carbs should be ingested throughout the course of the day, but they are particularly important during the times surrounding athletic activity. Before working out, carbs are important to bolster blood glucose and muscle glycogen stores. Athletes should consume a high carb meal about 3-4 hours before training. That means treating lunch as an important pre-training meal. In addition, a high carb snack should be taken about 2 hours before training (as real food, not a candy "power bar").

If the teenager is a, "scholastic athlete" who trains 1-2 hours a day at least 5 days a week, the post exercise meal becomes very important in replenishing diminished muscle glycogen. This glycogen is the primary fuel for the next day's workout. This meal is important in sparing muscle from post exercise breakdown. Maximize the build up of glycogen by providing this high carb meal with adequate protein from real food as soon as possible following the work out. This increases muscle strength and growth.

Adolescents are quick to accept the disinformation found is some "health" books, as in *Fit For Life* which claims without any scientific evidence that eating foods in certain combinations will render them indigestible or non-absorbable, or that "toxins" will form if certain foods are eaten together at different times of the day or night.

Read further about another dietary supplement called L-carnitine in PART 11: NUTRITION 101, following the Lipid Hypothesis. This so called "body building" compound produces trimethylamine-N-oxide (TMAO) in the gut and may lead to early onset atherosclerosis, heart attack and stroke.

When megadoses of a vitamin are recommended, beware of side effects. A vitamin given in doses so large that it is unlikely to have been obtained from one's natural diet may act more as a drug. By definition, a megavitamin is a vitamin given in a dose ten times the RDA or more. If there is a specific defect in a person's body chemistry limiting absorption of a vitamin or preventing normal amounts of vitamins from getting across cell walls into the body tissues, then megadose vitamins may be extremely helpful. Fortunately most of us do not have these problems.

If you still believe that a high saturated fat diet and cardiovascular disease is something that only adults should worry about, then listen to this: In the January 1997 issue of a prominent American Medical Journal it was shown how a high saturated fat diet is already at work causing artery blockage during early adolescence. Autopsies were performed on 1,079 men and 363 women between the ages of 15 and 34 who died accidentally. The researchers found dramatic differences in the severity of fatty deposits and lesions on the arteries of young people, depending on whether they smoked or ate diets rich in fat.

What is the typical teenage lunch or snack? A Big Mac, French fries and a chocolate shake provide 1000 calories, with 31 grams fat. (50% of these calories come from fat!) In addition the Big Mac has 960 mg of sodium, and that doesn't include what is on the French fries. There is negligible fiber and excess sugar. Many school cafeteria lunches are often as bad, and worse.

A simple and valid assessment of the nutritional needs of teenagers is that they are similar to those of other ages except for a greater need for calories. **If 65-70 % of calories are provided**

by complex carbohydrates and 10-12% by protein, most likely the necessary mineral, fiber, and vitamins will be automatically ingested.

Before moving on, a parental alert on Caffeine Energy drinks spiked with alcohol must be a part of "Nutrition News." These drinks have become extremely popular and are often used at teenage parties to mask to effects of the alcohol. Drinkers also drink beer with "Energy drinks" and drive under the influence of alcohol because they wrongfully perceive their judgment and reflexes are normal. The teenager (or adult) who had three alcoholic drinks and an energy drink is at the same level of intoxication as a person who had three drinks, but they think they're fine to drive.

There are special situations and needs during adolescence. No discussion on teenage nutrition is complete without some relevant information on iron.

Iron deficiency is one of the most widespread nutritional deficiency problems still seen in the United States. Although there is much written about other minerals and vitamins allegedly being in short supply in our diet, iron deficiency remains a real problem in infancy, adolescence and especially pregnancy.

When one thinks of iron deficiency, anemia is the problem that often comes to mind. **But depletion of body stores of iron causes many problems in the body long before anemia or low hemoglobin occurs.** By the time anemia is present, many other bodily changes have occurred. Vital metalloenzymes[70] are affected early, producing symptoms of irritability and poor appetite in children. Other behavioral changes such as pica, (eating dirt, soil, paint chips, etc.) and the craving for ice frequently occur. It has been suggested that alcoholism has occasionally resulted

[70] A *metalloenzyme* contains a metal as part of a protein catalyst. The role of trace minerals (metals) in enzymes and vitamins helps us understand the manner in which minerals participate in biologic processes and provides a fundamental basis in relating trace elements to health and disease.

from this ice craving since it is socially acceptable for adults to drink ice with alcoholic drinks. Allegedly the iron deficient compulsive ice eater gets habituated to the alcohol as well. Treatment with oral iron supplements results in the disappearance of the ice craving, poor appetite, and irritability usually within a week or two, and long before the anemia itself is corrected. Chronic fatigue is believed to be a relatively late symptom in iron deficiency, but decreased work performance has been found in people with even mild iron deficiency.

A simple hemoglobin test might appear normal, while iron deficiency may exist without symptoms. This is especially so during periods of rapid growth as during infancy, adolescence, and throughout the childbearing period in women. During these times when demand for iron for hemoglobin formation and muscle is increased, additional iron is needed in the diet. Especially at risk are premature infants and children 6 months to 3 years of age.

Researchers from Johns Hopkins Medical School reported in the British medical journal Lancet their study in which 700 teenage girls in Baltimore high schools were screened for iron deficiency. Scientists were looking for girls with low iron levels, but not low enough to cause anemia. This study's screening method differed from how most physicians screen for low iron levels. Usually physicians check a simple hemoglobin or hematocrit. If anemia is not found, it is assumed that iron levels are adequate. But anemia reflects only severe iron deficiency. Moderately low iron levels can exist without anemia.

The researchers found 73 girls, roughly 10%, who had low iron levels, but who had not yet developed iron deficiency anemia. These girls were then screened with several standardized tests to measure verbal learning skills and memory. The group of girls was then divided into two groups, making sure that both groups had similar levels of iron deficiency and similar test scores.

Half the girls were then treated with iron pills and the other were given identical placebos containing no iron. After eight weeks the girls were re-tested. The half that were given iron had higher blood iron levels and higher blood counts. This result was expected, but in addition this group also did significantly better on the verbal learning and memory tests. Eight weeks of iron therapy was effective in improving scores on these important measures of brain function in iron-deficient high school girls.

Regular aspirin users are also at high risk for iron deficiency. For these reasons public health-minded nutritionists have promoted fortification. Rather than relying on people to remember to take extra iron every day in pill form, iron has been added to flour and cereal. For those who prefer to get their iron from more natural sources, good ones are whole wheat, fish, poultry, figs, beans, asparagus, black strap molasses, dark green vegetables and extra lean meat. Prune juice, as mentioned earlier, is also an excellent source of iron. Cooking in iron pots and pans contributes a great deal of extra iron in the diet. The much fabled spinach[71], Popeye's ready source, has many milligrams of iron but the bio-availability[72] of this iron is poor because it is in the form of poorly absorbable iron oxalate. The same is true of the iron in egg yolk which is insoluble. Some foods decrease iron absorption. Bran and teas containing tannin[73] are two. (Coffee which contains no tannins, depresses absorption, but to a lesser degree). More than a quart of milk a day also contributes to iron deficiency.

Other foods increase iron absorption, particularly vitamin C rich foods, which counteract the effects of other iron inhibitors. Small amounts of animal protein (non-dairy) such as lean beef,

[71] Spinach is good for you. It is exceptionally high in beta carotene and folic acid.

[72] "Bioavailability "is that amount of a nutrient which the body can utilize or absorb when consumed.

[73] Tannin or tannic acid is what imparts the tan color to tea. This astringent vegetable compound also adds a constricting taste to your tongue and palate from strongly brewed tea .

breast of chicken, etc., added to a meal can increase iron absorption four fold. Vitamin C, however, is not an important enhancer of medicinal iron absorption.[74] This is important to remember, especially for pregnant women, who are often advised to take high doses of iron supplements. Taking a ferrous iron pill before breakfast insures excellent absorption.

Many people wish to take iron supplements because of the fact that absorption of iron from foods varies so greatly. In the ordinary diet 10-20mg of iron are ingested each day, but less than 10% of this is absorbed. The requirement for iron found in the RDA takes into account the low amount of iron actually absorbed from orally ingested iron. I tell my patients that in recommended doses iron is safe, but to be careful not to consume too much iron as a supplement[75] because in large amounts, it can cause abdominal discomfort and be toxic as well. Ferrous sulfate is a good supplement to take when a supplement is needed, as it is very well absorbed. Some "chelated iron" compounds sold because of their less irritating effect on the gut are often passed out in the stool without being utilized.

It is extremely rare for older teenage boys or young adult men to be anemic due to lack of iron. Anemia in adult men should always be thoroughly investigated for its cause. Taking iron tablets could hide and postpone early diagnosis or recognition of blood loss in the stool from colitis, polyps, or intestinal cancer.

---

[74] "Ferrous"iron is well absorbed. "Ferric"iron is the type of iron found in many vegetables. Vitamin C converts the poorly absorbed ferric iron to the more absorbable ferrous iron. Medicinal iron is "ferrous"that is, it's already in the "ferrous"state and therefore vitamin C will not further enhance its absorption.

[75] Be sure to put all pills or medicines locked or out of reach of climbing toddlers and young children. Iron poisoning remains one of the more common and often deadly poisonings in children.

RECOMMENDED DIETARY ALLOWANCES (RDA) FOR ELEMENTAL IRON ARE:

Elemental iron means available iron. For example:

HOW TO CALCULATE ELEMENTAL IRON FROM THE LABEL

Multiply the size (in milligrams) by the percentage of elemental iron in the iron form. Ferrous fumarate contains 33% elemental iron, Ferrous sulfate contains 20% elemental iron and ferrous gluconate contains 12% elemental iron.

Example: ferrous sulfate – 325 X .20 = 65mg elemental iron

Ferrous sulfate tablets that contain 325 mg of iron = 65 mg elemental or available iron.

Ferrous gluconate tablets that contain 325 mg of iron = 39 mg elemental or available iron.

Ferrous fumarate tablets that contain 200 mg of iron = 66 mg elemental or available iron.

Children's multivitamins with iron have very small amounts of elemental iron, typically 12-18 mg.

Infants

0-6 months 6 mg

6-12 months 10 mg

Children

Children 1-10 years 10 mg

Boys 11-18 years 12 mg

19+ 10 mg

Girls 11-18 years 15 mg

Women under 50 years 15 mg

Pregnant women 30 mg

Breastfeeding women 15 mg

Adult males and women over 50 years old 10 mg

One word of warning. Poison Centers have become increasingly alarmed about the number of iron poisonings in young children. **Iron poisonings kill more children under age six than any other substance** and most of these poisonings occur as a result of children accidentally ingesting iron tablets or prenatal vitamins. As few as ten tablets of 325mg. ferrous sulfate can be fatal to a child weighing less than 22 pounds. **Treatment of iron poisoning should not be delayed. If your child swallows iron pills, call your doctor and go to the emergency room right away!**

VITAMINS PREVENT BIRTH DEFECTS

Now I wish to fill you in on some important information about vitamins that is of practical importance to all teenage girls and all women capable of becoming pregnant.

Many vitamins and their derivatives are currently being used in the mainstream of medicine as a medicine. For example, pregnant women who take vitamins containing the recommended 0.4 mg of folate (folic acid) a day are 50% less likely to give birth to a child with neural tube defects (anencephaly-a baby born without a brain; or spine defects such as spina bifida.) It has been suggested that at least 1 mg of folate be given daily to all teenagers and women of childbearing age. Cleft lip and cleft palate are two more congenital birth defects that may be preventable by taking daily doses of folate before and during pregnancy in the very safe range of between 1mg and 10mg.[76] It is important that this vitamin be taken daily before a woman knows she is pregnant, because by the time of a missed period, it is usually too late and the damage has occurred. Each year approximately 2,500 infants are born with neural tube defects in America.

Folate is a water soluble B vitamin that is excreted in the urine and is not significantly stored in the body. It is needed to make DNA. If there is insufficient folate available to make this

[76] Any dose of folic acid above 1 mg daily needs to be taken only under medical supervision because a high dose of folic acid may mask the symptoms of undiagnosed pernicious anemia.

DNA, cell division halts. When the fetus is first developing, cell division is so rapid that body folic acid is quickly depleted unless replenished daily with a high green vegetable diet, orange juice, and /or with folate supplementation. Once the critical period of organ formation is passed, it is too late. Additional folate will not correct the problem once the facial, brain, or spinal cord defect has occurred. Most pregnancies are unplanned, and this is especially true with adolescents. That is why it is so important to give the daily supplements to all girls and women of childbearing ages and not to totally rely on dietary intake of folate.

Fortunately folic acid is an extremely safe vitamin. The required dosage of folate can be furnished by certain breakfast cereals and leafy green vegetables as well as fresh orange juice, but a supplement is recommended for those who are at high risk.

Folic acid, by the way, has recently been thought to protect the heart and was being used as a dietary medicine to help prevent the events that lead to heart attacks and stroke. Doctors had speculated that folic acid may improve heart health because people with B-vitamin deficiencies often have high blood levels of the amino acid homocysteine, a marker of inflammation that has been linked to increased risk of heart disease, but a large new study suggests that even though folic acid lowers blood homocysteine, heart attacts and strokes are not lowered. Homocysteine remains to be a marker for inflammation, however, the blood test CRP (C Reactive Protein) has replaced it as a better marker of inflammation. More on the "Inflammation Hypothesis" as a cause of cardiovascular disease can be found in PART II following " The Lipid Hypothesis."

Although the water soluble B vitamins are usually safe even when taken in excess of the RDA, beware of the possible side effects of large doses of any vitamins. There are times when "more" is not better, and it is the healthy teenager who is most vulnerable to the hype that more is better. For example, **the fat**

soluble vitamin A is linked to birth defects when taken in amounts above the RDA. Even as little as the amount contained in two or three multivitamin pills, or anything more than 10,000 international units a day of vitamin A may be dangerous to the developing fetus. One of every 57 babies born to women who had taken more than 10,000 units of vitamin A will have a birth defect as a result. The problems involved malformations of the face, head, heart, and nervous system. Therefore, to be safe, check your vitamin bottles and be sure that the vitamin A levels do not exceed 5000 units, the current recommended dietary allowance (RDA). I personally believe that the inclusion of vitamin A in over the counter multivitamins in the USA is not only unnecessary, but a public health danger. This vitamin is a well documented teratogen (a substance that causes malformations in the unborn child) and to have it incorporated with a prenatal vitamin seems to be a poor decision, especially in a country where vitamin A deficiency is at worst, marginal. (Vitamin A deficiency is common in undeveloped countries because of poverty and ignorance.) The less toxic beta-carotene might be considered as a more logical replacement because beta carotene is the safe, non toxic form of vitamin A, even when ingested in large amounts.

Supplement use in general has soared since the 1970's. But unless you are pregnant or have specific deficiencies, eating a healthy and balanced diet remains the best way to ensure that you're getting all the essential vitamins. Supper-supplementation does not have a role.

PART II

▲ ▲ ▲

NUTRITION 101

THE CHEMICALS OF LIFE

▲ ▲ ▲

This primer offers the basics for understanding what infants, children and adolescents need nutritionally, and what foods will fulfill those needs. Without a basic understanding of the chemicals of nutrition (carbohydrates, protein, fats, fiber, vitamins and minerals), the important objective of ensuring nutritional well being could be easily clouded. A knowledge of how dietary chemicals are utilized by the body is important in determining how much of these foods are needed for health and for the restoration of body tissue in stress and disease. For this reason, these chapters on are included. Readers should keep in mind that research is constantly adding to our knowledge of nutrition and therefore new information may alter some of the information presented in this book. We must always try to keep an open mind and be prepared to change our beliefs when new, scientifically collected data warrant it.

The much abbreviated information that follows is a crash course in the basics of nutrition. It will help you read food labels and what's between the lines of these labels. It will make you much smarter about food; and if you act on what you learn here, it will help you and your family become healthier.

ENERGY

Our bodies require a certain amount of fuel to operate efficiently and the fuel we run on is **energy derived from calories. Many people don't know that a source of energy is nothing more than a source of calories.** The amount of calories we need depends primarily upon our height, weight, age, and the type and amount of activity in which we normally engage. If you take in more calories than you can use, your remarkable body converts the excess into body fat and stores it for possible future use. It takes about 3500-4000 calories to produce a pound of body fat.

Calories are delivered to the body as sugars derived from carbohydrates, proteins and fats. Metabolism is the means by which energy is made available to the body. The basal metabolic rate of a person is the amount of calories needed to "run" the body at rest (during sleep). Added to that is the amount of energy needed (calories) to fuel "normal" daily activity and the calories needed to maintain weight and growth. A sedentary person uses fewer calories (energy) than the one in perpetual motion. Infants and adolescents also need many extra calories because these ages are times of rapid growth. After age 35 or 40, many adults who do not exercise need fewer calories to maintain weight. In addition, many adults begin to move more slowly (more efficiently?) and, therefore, find themselve putting on excess weight while consuming the same amount of calories they ate during their more youthful years. If an adult consumes a mere 25 calories a day in excess of need, in 365 days that would add up to about 9000 calories or a two pound weight gain. If this habit continues, in ten years that would translate to a 20 pound weight gain! This is the plight of many once slender young adults, but it also helps to explain why slow moving children gain weight so easily, when compared to the skinny child who is in constant motion and consumes twice the calories.

Too many calories are a major cause of an expanding waistline, especially if those calories are mostly from fructose or HFCS.

CARBOHYDRATES

▲ ▲ ▲

The following extremely important information on the biochemistry of foods will help you understand these fundamental concepts and appreciate how fuzzy nutritional notions can direct you to poor nutritional and dietary choices.

The **carbohydrates** are called **saccharides** (compounds made up of sugar). The simplest are the **monosaccharides** which are also known as simple sugars. Examples of simple sugars are **glucose**, or blood sugar; **fructose**, or fruit sugar, the predominant sugar in honey; and **galactose**, a simple milk sugar. All sugars contain 4 calories per gram.

When two **monsaccharides** or simple sugars combine chemically, they form a double sugar, called a **disaccharide**. **Sucrose** (table sugar), **lactose** (milk sugar) and maltose (malt sugar) are examples of the most common dietary disaccharides.

The more complex carbohydrates are known as polysaccharides. Their molecules are composed of combinations of monosaccharides or sugar molecules and are very large. Examples are starch, glycogen (animal starch), and cellulose. The complex carbohydrate, starch, is found chiefly in plants such as corn, rice, potatoes, yams, and grains. Cellulose forms the cell walls of plants. Cellulose and starch are made up of simple sugars linked together. The linkages are different enough to make starch digestible but cellulose indigestible.

Another class of complex carbohydrates, consisting of "polymers" of monosaccharides, are the **oligosaccharides**. Oligosaccharides may prove useful as additives to nutritional products such as infant formulas and adult supplements because of their immune properties. Human breast milk, for example, contains 25 different oligosaccharides, which probably function as natural anti-infective agents.[77] There appears to be a correlation between the oligosaccharide content in breast milk and immunity at birth. These oligosaccharides may play an important role in protecting the newborn with an as yet underdeveloped immune system, and may be the newborns first line of defense against infections.

*Oligosaccharide anti-infective agents. Lancet. April 13, 1996; 347.

The **simple sugars** are absorbed very rapidly from the digestive tract while complex carbohydrates break down slowly during the digestive process, eventually being reduced to the simple sugars. They are then absorbed into the blood stream in their simple form and converted into energy (calories) for the body to "burn" as fuel for activity or stored as fat for later use.

From this you can understand the theory of giving juices to provide "instant energy" or the before game carbohydrate-loading meals of athletes as a source of "slow release" energy or fuel during major competitions.

Here is some practical information about sugar and carbohydrates. The sugar bowl on your kitchen counter is only the tip of the iceberg. There are hundreds of forms of sugar hidden in our diet. Punch, apple and orange juice, energy drinks, fresh fruit, ice cream, hot and dry cereals, pies, donuts, cookies, candy, muffins, chili, pizza, Jello, hot dogs, bacon, ham, salami and cold cuts, stuffing, breads, soups, mayonnaise, catsup, salad

[77] "Oligosaccharide anti-infective agent." Lancet. April 13, 1996: 347

dressing, sweetened yogurt, canned vegetables, beans, and virtually all frozen foods to mention a few.

Besides refined cane and beet sugars (common table sugar sucrose), there is refined fructose, which is similar to other table sugars. Advocates of fructose claim that because it is one and a half times as sweet as sucrose, people will use less. Fructose as are all carbohydrates provides 4 calories per gram, but it has special properties that allow it to be metabolized in a different way. We now understand that high fructose corn syrup (HFCS) and fructose is harmful. This will be discussed in more detail later. This widely used alternative sugar and corn syrup is used as an inexpensive sweetener in many sodas and baked goods.

The average American consumed about 110-130 pounds of sugar per year in 1998. In 2012 that number is 150 pounds of sugar per year! It is estimated that the average American now consumes 22-28 teaspoons of added sugars a day. This comes mostly from high-fructose corn syrup and sucrose.

This represents 18-20% of calories consumed daily in a typical American diet, and that doesn't include the sugar calories from fresh fruit and fruit juices. My recommendation is that total carbohydrate calories should amount to about 65% of calories consumed, and most of these should be from complex carbohydrate. When 20% of calories are contributed by sugar, 30% by fat, 15% by protein what's left is a mere 35% of calories available from complex carbohydrates. This high sugar consumption displaces minerals, vitamins and fiber found in complex carbohydrates. The lost fiber content from these foods promotes constipation and indirectly contributes to other diseases such as diverticulitis[78], and obesity.

Although there is no RDA for sugar, the American Heart Association suggested a limit of no more than 100 calories a day for adult women and no more than 150 calories a day for men.

[78] Diverticulitis is an inflammation of a diverticulum (a tubular sac or outpouching) of the colon.

Other sugars used commercially are molasses, maple syrup, honey, dextrose, lactose, levulose, and the "alcoholic sugars" mannitol, maltitol and sorbitol.

Nutritious foods such as dried apples, apricots, and prunes, as well as fresh fruit are all high in sugars. These sugars are also sucrose and fructose, but they are combined with other nutrients such as minerals, vitamins, and fiber. Sucrose and fructose when in refined forms such as juice, or table sugar, whether white or brown, have been stripped of the fiber content and much of their mineral and vitamin content. In addition, these **refined** simple carbohydrates don't fill you up as do the high fiber, low fat complex carbohydrates. Because complex carbohydrates are bulky, you fill up before overeating.

Most of us have experienced the effect from drinking these simple sugars as a "pick-up" when we are tired or hungry. Because they are rapidly absorbed into the bloodstream, the body responds by pouring out insulin to lower this rise in blood sugar. This causes the blood sugar to quickly fall, often at a level below the original amount. Hunger returns along with "the shakes" as body adrenaline is released to counteract the insulin. Besides this rollercoaster effect, there is evidence that the increase in insulin promotes the dietary sugar to be converted into fat. It seems as though it is the fructose sugar that is most harmful to health.

Children and adults who consume fructose, the main sugar in sodas, are more likely to have increased belly fat, called visceral fat. Visceral fat is fat that invades the liver, muscles and around the gut causing the unwanted "pot belly" sometimes referred to as beer belly. There is a relationship between a large belly, insulin resistance, diabetes, liver and heart disease.

Sugar promotes tooth decay especially when consumed between meals as a sticky candy, in raisins or pastry. Behavior problems such as hyperactivity have been attributed to a high sugar diet, but most studies have not substantiated this association.

The contagious enthusiasm of a birthday party or "free time" at school may be the real culprit rather than sugar. It has become much in vogue to blame misbehavior, learning problems, etc., on refined sugar. I suspect in many cases this may be an attractive escape from the responsibility of improving one's home and school structure. Class size and structure may have more to do with "hyperactivity," and "attentiveness" than diet. Sugar may be a factor in some children. A parent might swear that when her child is exposed to a particular food, he or she would become hyperactive. My suggestion is that a prudent approach would be to avoid the suspected offending food. Skin, blood testing, or sublingual testing has not proved to be of much value.

ADHD is a condition that is increasing. There are multiple factors such as family history, genetics, diet, and many other unknowns. Dr. Benjamin Feingold, a pediatric allergist, suspected that salicylates, a naturally occurring compound present in many fruits, some vegetables and a number of other foods, plus artificial colors and artificial flavors are causes of hyperactivity. The Feingold Diet was very popular in the 1970's. It eliminates essentially all manufactured baked goods, luncheon meats, ice cream, powdered pudding, candies, soft drinks and canned fruit drinks. It also eliminates toothpaste, cough drops and mouthwash. Does this work? It is estimated that about 2-3% of the ADHD population may be helped by this diet.

HFCS, fructose and simple sugar, also contributes to sleep apnea, arthritis, high blood pressure, stroke, and increased risk of cancers of the colon, breast, prostate, and uterus.

Like fats, sugar has an important place in nutrition when consumed in small amounts. What do I mean by, "small?" In 2009, reported in the American Journal of Clinical Nutrition 89: 1037,– 88, 000 nurses were followed for 24 years. Those nurses who consumed at least two sugar-sweetened drinks a day had a

35% higher risk of heart attack than those who drank less than one a month. Keep that in mind the next time you succumb to your child's pleadings for a Coke.

THE FOLLOWING IS A LIST OF SIMPLE CARBOHYDRATES

Agave	Evaporated cane juice
Sucrose	Corn syrup
High Fructose Corn Syrup (HFCS)	Maple syrup
Glucose	Molasses
Fructose	Honey
Dextrose	Syrup
Invert sugar	Corn sweetener
Brown sugar	Orange juice concentrate
Grape juice concentrate	Apple juice concentrate
Table sugar	Raw sugar

EXAMPLES OF FOODS HIGH IN SIMPLE CARBOHYDRATES

Berries	Bananas
Oranges	Grapefruit
Apricots	Apples
Melons	Orange juice
Grapefruit juice	Apple juice
Apricot nectar	Peach nectar
Kool Aid	Lemonade
Energy drinks	Hi-C
Tang	Hard candy
Coca-Cola	Soda

FOODS CONTAINING COMPLEX CARBOHYDRATES (STARCH AND CELLULOSE)

LEGUMES

Peas Beans Garbanzos Peanuts String Beans

TUBERS

Carrots Yams Potato

CRUCIFERS

Broccoli, Chard , Cauliflower, Cabbage, Bok Choy, Brussels Sprouts, Broccolini[79]

OTHER VEGETABLES

Lettuce, Celery, Asparagus, Eggplant, Cucumber, Onion, Garlic, Tomato

GRAINS

Rice, Wild Rice, Wheat Buckwheat, Rye, Oats, Barley, Quinoa, Corn Popcorn Millet, Triticale.

79 Check out this new vegetable. It is a cross of broccoli and Chinese kale. It looks like a streamlined broccoli with an asparagus-like stem and tastes like sweet broccoli. It is lighter, sweeter, more tender and fresher tasting than broccoli.

The foods containing complex carbohydrates have a small percentage of fat and protein in addition to starch and cellulose, the indigestible cell walls of plants. Remember that when you eat rice, corn, potato, or pasta, you are not eating pure starch. For example buckwheat (if you roast buckwheat before you boil it, you've got kasha) is fiber rich and high in copper and magnesium while wild rice has more zinc than any other grain. Barley is a good source of fiber and iron, while brown rice is the only rice that contains vitamin E. These foods contain significant protein with minimal fat, as long as you don't douse them with butter, margarine, oil, or cream. If you must use a "flavor enhancer" use an herbal non-fat sour cream or something similar to "I Can't Believe It's Not Butter." Fresh salsa is another delicious and nutritious topping.

THE GLYCEMIC INDEX

The glycemic index refers to the degree blood sugar (glucose) increases after eating a single food. Foods that are absorbed quickly into the bloodstream have high glycemic indexes; those with sugars that are absorbed slowly have low glycemic indexes. The glycemic index ranks foods on a 100 point scale, with 100 being the fastest rate of absorption.

A number of factors influence glycemic responses to food, including the amount of carbohydrate, type of sugar, nature of starch (amylase, amylopectin, resistant starch) cooking and food processing, food form, and other food components such as fat and natural substances that slow digestion. Examples of these are lectins, phytates, tannins, and starch-protein and starch-lipid combinations. Most of us consume high glycemic index foods along with the above foods, thus making the glycemic index less helpful.

It is useful to know the glycemic index of a particular food, but it should not be the only criterion for including or neglecting it in the diet. Cutting back on all foods with high glycemic indexes would cause you to avoid many foods that are healthy in other ways, including carrots (glycemic index of 71), sweet potatoes (glycemic index of 54, and brown rice (glycemic index of 55).[80]

The current validated methods use glucose as the reference food, giving it a glycemic index value of 100 by definition.

Glycemic index of foods are commonly interpreted as follows:

Low GI	55 or less
Medium GI	56-69
High GI	70 and above

Tables of Glycemic Index, Human Nutrition Unit, Department of Biochemistry, University of Sydney.

Food (ranked high to low)	Glycemic Index
Potato	90
Corn Flakes	77
Donut	76
Bagel, plain	72
Ice Cream	61
Cheese pizza	60
Oatmeal cookies	54
Banana	53
Chocolate	49
Apple	36
Yogurt, low-fat with fruit and sugar	33
Milk, skim	32

80

All-bran cereal	30
Kidney beans	27
Milk, whole	27
Yogurt, low-fat with artificial sweetener	14

PROTEINS

▲ ▲ ▲

Proteins differ from carbohydrates and fats chemically in that they contain nitrogen. The proteins of our bodies are **composed of twenty-two amino acids, in varying combinations.** Of these, eight can't be made by our bodies and are therefore called **essential amino acids.** These amino acids must be obtained in adequate amounts from the food we eat. They are tryptophan, leucine, isoleucine, lysine, valine, threonine, phenylalanine and methionine. All eight amino acids must be present in order for a protein to be nutritionally complete. **Proteins that contain the essential amino acids in adequate quantities are called complete proteins.** Examples are egg white, fish, meat, poultry and certain vegetables, such as soybean and peanut.

Our bodies digest protein to form amino acids. Amino acids are necessary for growth, repair, and maintenance of our body tissues. We need a basic minimum of protein to remain in "positive nitrogen balance." That is, we need to have enough protein intake to balance what our body wears out or excretes. If you are in "negative nitrogen balance," it means that you are excreting more nitrogen (protein) than you are consuming. Your body must then obtain nitrogen by breaking down your muscles and the cells. This is extremely unhealthy and is called starvation!

How digestible a protein is, especially a plant protein, determines how much of its amino acids are actually available to our bodies. Whole proteins must be digested to amino acids before being absorbed into the bloodstream from the intestines. The term "biological value" is used to describe proteins as complete or incomplete. Complete proteins of high biological value are found in meats, egg white, fish, poultry, edamame (fresh soybeans), and nuts. The proteins that do not supply the essential amino acids, or else supply inadequate amounts, are known as incomplete or inadequate. They are usually of vegetable origin and that is why vegetarians should eat a greater quantity or variety of plant proteins. Having said this, I will reiterate that protein deficiency is not a nutritional problem in America. Nutritionists point out the need for increased protein intake during periods of the life cycle when rapid growth takes place. These are infancy, teenage years and pregnancy. However, protein from meat intake in America is in such excess that we see more of the toxic effects of too much animal protein than protein deficiency.

For example, infants are occasionally fed cowmilk which has 20% protein, far in excess of the more nutritional 7% protein of human breast milk. Adolescents often take protein drinks believing that this will increase their muscle bulk and strength. This poor nutrition is not only unnecessary, but potentially dangerous. Too much protein also results in increased loss of minerals, such as calcium.

The RDA for protein for a growing male adolescent who is tall and well developed is 56 grams a day. For those nutritionists who refer to the RDA as a guide, use caution. **The National Research Council suggests that a diet should not be considered inadequate if it does not meet the recommended levels.**

For those individuals not in a rapid growth phase or not pregnant, 10% of calories is sufficient protein. Pregnant and breastfeeding mothers need extra protein but not nearly as much as some nutritionists recommend. The RDA suggests 74 grams of protein for a pregnant woman and 64 grams for a breastfeeding mother. Remember, this is a very high value and may be extremely inappropriate and excessive for a 5' tall 108 pound woman. For this reason it is more accurate to calculate protein needs using height and body build plus percent of total calories needed, as well as state of health. Few parents will tax their math skill to determine protein needs, and indeed, they shouldn't. In the real world, nobody does this. **I do not want to stress numbers,** since they will soon be forgotten and are irrelevant to the shopper, who shops for food, and should **rely on principles,** such as buying fresh produce, whole grains, avoiding high fructose corn syrup (HFCS) cakes, cookies and sugary drinks along with **high saturated fat protein foods.** The at risk population for protein deficiency is the teenage girl on a diet soda and candy bar diet or the pregnant teenager. These children need special attention and nutritional counseling.

Since 1983, I have worked as a pediatrician in many Central and South American countries as well as in Asia and Africa with an organization, Rotaplast International, Inc. My responsibility was to examine each child who needed a cleft lip or palate surgery to make certain the child was healthy enough to undergo surgery plus supervised post-operative and convalescent care.

I will never forget the first time I witnessed the devastating effects of protein deficiency. We just completed reconstructing this beautiful six month old infant's cleft lip.[81] She was slightly

[81] Cleft lip is a condition where a child is born with incomplete closure of

anemic. What I didn't realize was that the infant's poor and uneducated parents were feeding their daughter an infant formula they made with a little milk formula, and extended with mostly cooked corn meal. This is a common practice, since commercial baby formula is expensive, and mothers are not encouraged to breastfeed. Corn is an incomplete protein because it does not contain the essential amino acid tryptophan. As a result, the child was protein deficient, and because I was unaware of her diet, I permitted the surgery to take place. When the baby's sutures were removed at the usual time healing had not occurred, and the beautiful repair fell apart. That moment was the beginning of my interest in nutrition.

Inadequate intake of essential amino acids over an extended period of time causes "protein starvation" and the protein deficiency disease, kwashiorkor results. Kwashiorkor is an African name that describes affected children with characteristic red hair, swollen bodies and potbellies. I've seen kwashiorkor many times since that episode in Honduras, and other developing countries where poor mothers feed their children formula made from corn instead of breastfeeding. This is a third world disease and is extremely rare in the United States where over-consumption of protein is the rule.

If one is a vegetarian, or especially vegan, who does not eat any egg white, dairy or fish, the selection of foods must be more careful.

True malnutrition does occur in the United States, but it is usually because of ignorance, or a psychotic parent or caretaker. In Marin County, Northern California, there was such a family

---

the lip. This condition, called "harelip" in the past is usually repaired by plastic surgeons before the infant is six months old. Cleft palate, refers to incomplete closure of the palate, leaving a hole in the roof of the mouth. If this defect is not closed before the child is one year of age, difficult to correct, life-long speech problems often occur. The congenital defects may be genetic (run in families) or may be caused by environmental or nutritional factors, such as insufficient folic acid in the diet. Taking folic acid <u>before</u> pregnancy occurs protects against many types of cleft lip and cleft palate.

who provided a low fat, low carbohydrate, low protein vegan diet to their five children. When one died, an autopsy revealed the baby to have severe rickets.

The other children were inspected by CPS (Child Protective Services). The children were found to be developmentally delayed, with boney malformations, and emaciation. They were immediately transferred to UCSF Medical Center and were found to have advanced severe rickets due to extremely poor nutrition with lack of vitamin D in the diet plus little sun exposure.

THE RDA

The RDA are "estimates of amounts of essential nutrients each person in a healthy population must consume in order to provide reasonable assurance that the physiologic needs of all will be met." This is a public health concept, according to Dr. Alfred E. Harper, past chairman of the committee on RDA. "The underlying premise," he states, "is that, since the requirements of individuals are not known, the recommendations must be **high enough** to meet the needs of those with the highest requirements. For essential nutrients, therefore, **the RDA must exceed the requirements of most members of the population."**

FATS (LIPIDS)

▲ ▲ ▲

Although fat is the name often applied to all lipids, the broad category of chemicals with greasy properties, such as fat (triglycerides), fatty acids, and cholesterol are classified as lipids. The chemical composition of fats is similar to carbohydrate, but one gram of fat produces a hefty 9 calories, over twice the calories obtained from one gram of protein or sugar.

The fats in fatty tissue (adipose tissue) are called triglycerides. Triglycerides are one of the three parts of cholesterol in the body: low-density lipoproteins (LDL), high-density lipoproteins (HDL) and triglycerides. When we eat calories in excess, particularly carbohydrates, the body transforms these carbohydrates into glucose. Glucose is then used by the body for energy. However, not all glucose is used. These forms are transferred to the liver where glucose is converted into glycogen ("animal glucose"), which is then stored in the muscles. Excess glycogen is moved back from the muscles to the liver and the glycogen becomes triglycerides, which are stored as fats or in the blood stream. The triglycerides in the bloodstream are thick and fatty in nature. This means the blood can more easily clot and cause a blockage in your bloodstream. This can lead to dangerous side effects, such as inflammation, heart attack or stroke. As you can see, it is important for good health to keep your triglyceride levels low. A diet high in refined sugar, especially fructose, raises triglycerides

This body fat (triglycerides) breaks down into glycerol and three fatty acids. **Glycerol** can then be converted into sugar and used as body fuel. The **fatty acids** come in many different lengths and levels of saturation. **Saturated fatty acids** are opaque at room temperature and are mainly derived from animal sources. Examples of foods which contain predominantly saturated fatty acids are, whole and 2% milk, cream, ice cream, cheese, butter, beef, lamb, pork, coconut, coconut oil, and palm oil. **Fatty acids (fats) that are liquid at room temperature are usually more "unsaturated." Monounsaturated** fats, (olive oil, canola oil, avocado) seem to be healthier than saturated fat. When monounsaturated fat **replaces saturated fat in the diet**, it may have a blood cholesterol lowering effect (lowers LDL cholesterol levels). But can olive oil be used in baking? Some olive oils, such as regular, highly processed olive oil, have a very mild flavor in contrast to extra-virgin and virgin varieties. Olive oil may be used in place of butter or other solid fats in the baking of cakes, cookies, muffins and quick breads. It doesn't work well for pastries or crusts, because olive or any other oil saturates the flour and makes the finished product dense instead of light and flaky. **Polyunsaturated** fats (soybean oil, corn oil, safflower oil) appear to cause less damage to arterial walls than saturated fats, unless they are hydrogenated to make them a solid fat such as stick margarine or Crisco. **Hydrogenated polyunsaturated** fats contain what is called "trans" fat and are more damaging to your arteries than saturated animal fat such as bacon grease, butter or cream. Trans fats[82] are found in foods such as French fries, Oreo cookies, pie

---

[82] Minimize the use of vegetable oils that have hydrogenated or processed to make them stable and solid at room temperature. Hydrogenated fat contains significant amounts of "trans-fats." Trans-fat is found in processed cookies,

crusts, chicken pot pie crust, (one of the worst foods!), potato chips, and many other foods that may be labeled, "cholesterol-free." Fish fried in melted Crisco or stick margarine[83] along with Tatter-Tot and Chicken nuggets may be loaded with artery clogging trans fat. Look at the Nutrition Facts label. Trans-fats are now required to be listed on the Nutrition Facts label. Many fast food restaurants have recently removed trans fats from their cooking oil. Foods can call themselves "trans-fats free" even if they contain up to a gram of trans fats per serving. If a food contains partially hydrogenated oils, it contains trans fats.

The best way to reduce your triglycerides is to lower simple carbohydrates in the diet. Another way to reduce triglyceride levels is to consume more fatty fish, such as salmon or trout. Taking a daily supplement or fish oil also reduces triglyceride levels.

In addition, oils are available in two forms: **combined oil** is in the seed or fruit (avocado)[84] as grown. **Free oil** can be expressed, bottled and sold. Corn oil, safflower and sunflower seed oils are all free oils. Combined oil has the vitamins, minerals, fiber and other nutrients. To obtain free oil from corn, many kernels must be pressed to get one ounce.

---

chips, cake and crackers, in deep fried foods such as doughnuts, margarine and shortening. The amount of trans-fat now appears on the "Nutritional Facts" food labels, but watch out for "partially-hydrogenated oils" in package ingredient lists. This is a hidden source of trans-fat.

[83] A relatively new margarine, marketed as Benecol, contains a plant substance (a stanol ester) that prevents cholesterol absorption and can be used as a spread as well as for cooking. This margarine is being promoted as a natural cholesterol lowering food. It may turn out to be the margarine of choice if all the early studies on this product prove to be true. Recent studies suggest that there is insufficient stanol in one serving of Benecol to be effective in achieving a lowering effect.

[84] Avocados are high in monounsaturated fats, and are believed to be less harmful than saturated or trans fats. But beware of eating too much guacamole because calories do count. Don't let "good" fat or the "low fat" label give you a license to pig out. There is a trend toward overeating driven by the assumption that we can eat all we want as long as it's low in saturated fat.

Cholesterol is a lipid or fat-like substance which is found in all animal meat, whole and low fat milk, cheese, butter, liver, sweetbreads, eggs, shrimp, crab, and shell fish. Cholesterol is not found in any vegetables. All those "cholesterol free" advertisements stamped on vegetable oils and margarine are deceptive in that they suggest "healthy," or that somehow the cholesterol was removed. As you will learn, trans fat, and saturated fats are far more artery clogging (atherogenic) than cholesterol. Fats in combination with cholesterol are especially atherogenic (bacon & eggs; lobster dipped in butter, or melted stick margarine). Boiled shrimp dipped in a non-fat cocktail sauce is a delicious low fat dish and as long as the shrimp is not sautéed or fried, its small amount of cholesterol is of little nutritional consequence.

We have learned in recent years that there are various types of cholesterol, defined in terms of the types of protein they are associated with in the body. Since cholesterol, in pure form, is insoluble in water and blood, it tends to hook up with proteins forming what is called lipoprotein. Lipoprotein is a fat that has linked with a protein. This is the form in which cholesterol travels in the blood stream.

The body is able to make cholesterol, mainly in the liver, intestinal mucosa (lining), and various body tissues. **Some ends up as low density lipoprotein (LDL) and some as high density lipoprotein (HDL).** It is primarily the LDL of cholesterol that is most artery clogging (atherogenic) and lead to atherosclerotic vascular disease (heart attacks, strokes, blocked arteries) and that is why **LDL is often referred to as the "bad cholesterol." High density lipoproteins (HDL)** actually appears to protect against the build up of artery clogging "plaques." HDL (high density lipoproteins) provides a mechanism for removal of excess cholesterol from the bloodstream. **HDL cholesterol is often referred to as the "good cholesterol."** Aerobic exercise, and substitution of monounsaturated fats for saturated fats raises the good HDL's. (Use olive oil or canola oil instead of butter, margarine, shortening, lard, coconut oils, or hydrogenated polyunsaturated fats).

Small amounts of fats in our diet are important because they contribute a necessary source of flavor. Dietary fat has essential physiologic roles. It delays emptying time of the stomach, thereby delaying the onset of hunger, stores energy, and is part of every cell membrane. In the gut certain vitamins are absorbed from fats. Cholesterol is important in bile formation (needed for digestion), adrenal, and sex hormones, and has many other important functions such as brain growth. The body can manufacture cholesterol and most fatty acids. Fatty acids not synthesized by our body must be obtained from our food. These are called **essential fatty acids**. The three fatty acids known to be essential for complete nutrition of infants, children and adults are **linoleic acid**, (also referred to as **omega-6 fatty acids**), **linolenic acid**, (referred to as **omega-3 fatty acids**) and **arachiodonic acid** (another omega-6 fatty acid). **The reason essential fatty acid deficiency is extremely rare is that diets as low as eight percent fat carry no risk of fat deficiency disease!**

There are some fatty acids found in fish, such as salmon, called **DHA** (decosahexaenoic acid) and **EPA** (eicosapentaenoic acid) are anti-inflammatory and that may provide a protective effect against the formation of artery blocking cholesterol plaques, and seem to be especially important for brain development during infancy. DHA is found in breast milk and it has recently been added to commercial baby formula because of its reported IQ enhancing effect. My mother was correct when she referred to fish as "brain food."

It is common to hear supposedly well-informed individuals announce their "low cholesterol levels" as a badge of honor. **(Normal healthy cholesterol ranges between 125mg to 165mg).** How naive it is for adults or children to assume that they can consume all the fried eggs, ice cream, Tater tots, sausage or hot dogs, potato chips and French fries they desire because they are "thin" or their cholesterol level is low. A diet high in saturated fats, salt and highly refined carbohydrate (sugars), regardless of one's blood cholesterol level, will make one more likely to develop bowel cancer[85], hypertension, gallbladder disease, chronic constipation, and adult onset diabetes (type II).

Adult onset diabetes is often referred to as Non-Insulin-Dependent Diabetes Mellitus or Type II. People with diabetes have difficulty removing the sugar or glucose from their blood. After we digest a meal, glucose (blood sugar) is produced. In response, **the pancreas then secretes insulin,** a hormone that enables glucose to pass into the cells, where it is stored as fat or burned as body fuel. **In adult onset diabetes, insulin is produced, but it loses its effectiveness** and is unable to adequately remove enough glucose from the bloodstream. Overweight and under active people who have a familial history of diabetes seem to more readily develop this **insulin resistance** or Type II diabetes. Exercise and weight loss help prevent the onset of this type of diabetes, which close to 95% of diabetics have.

Type I Diabetes is often referred to as Juvenile Diabetes. **In Type I Diabetes there is little or no insulin** because most of the insulin producing pancreatic cells have been destroyed by something, perhaps a virus. It is unclear what this or these agents are, but the illness is different than the more prevalent Type II.

In insulin resistant Type II Diabetes, a diet high in saturated fat and refined sugar is especially dangerous because these diabetics are at great risk for developing atherosclerosis and a heart attack. In an effort to keep the body's blood sugar normal, lots of insulin is secreted. As a side effect, the body's triglycerides rise (blood fat), LDL's ("bad cholesterol") rise and the HDL's ("good cholesterol") fall. Heart disease begins along with stroke, kidney failure, and blindness...all part of the disease. Most adults can prevent or delay the onset of these complications by following the dietary advice given in this book. By getting more exercise, eating less saturated fat and protein, increasing complex

[85] In spite of many wild claims found in best selling nutrition books, no scientific cause and effect relationship has been established between diet and breast cancer.

carbohydrates and fiber, avoiding sugary foods and drinks, you will not only extend your life, you will improve life's quality and better enjoy your children and grandchildren.

Higher consumption of sugar-sweetened beverages by children 12-18 years old is associated with the consumption of foods that are a top source of saturated fat, such as pizza, cakes/cookies/pies, fried potatoes, and sweets!

THE LIPID HYPOTHESIS[86]

In 1904, the German scientist Felix Marchaud proposed the name, "**atherosclerosis**" for an arterial disease characterized by obstructive patches, **called plaques**, within arteries. These atheromatous arteries[87] contained up to 20 times as much cholesterol as normal arteries. By 1912, Dr. James Herrick clearly identified and described how heart attacks are associated with atherosclerosis of the coronary arteries. That dietary saturated fats and cholesterol as found in animal protein could predictably increase a person's serum cholesterol was first established in the 1950's and 1960's. Much evidence now exists that an elevated serum concentration of cholesterol is a causal factor in the development of arterial atherosclerosis and coronary heart disease. **Even a modest elevation to as little as 200mg can be significant in forming these obstructing plaques.** There are reputable scientists today that criticize this hypothesis because 100% evidence is not yet available. These nutritionists have not accepted the lipid hypothesis despite the growing body of evidence that supports it. Statements made publicly and widely disseminated by TV, radio, and the press have added to the confusion. The "cholesterol controversy" or more appropriately, the "saturated fat controversy," is being kept alive by special interest groups that are more concerned about the health of the beef, poultry and

86 The German Pathologist Rudolf Virchow described in 1856

87 Arteries that are filled with fatty cholesterol plaques.

dairy industries. Similar "controversy" over salt as a major cause of high blood pressure is now being disseminated by the major salt using, processed and frozen food industry.

Just as the tobacco industry has not succeeded in convincing intelligent adults that cigarettes are really harmless and non-addicting, those who suggest cholesterol, fats or high salt intake are not related to heart disease offer equally flimsy reasoning. Enough convincing evidence exists to strongly and safely recommend that for continued good health a diet should be low in fats, cholesterol, simple sugars, and salt. It should contain moderate amounts of protein, be high in complex carbohydrate, and fiber rich foods.

In addition to saturated fats, trans fats, cholesterol, and sugar, there are other players that contribute to the development of atherosclerosis. There are genetic or familial factors, antioxidants, and possibly infectious agents[88], such as viruses or other microbes that may initially damage the lining of arterial walls, thus setting in motion the formation of cholesterol laden atherosclerotic plaques. Particularly intriguing is the growing evidence pointing toward the role of germs or microorganisms, called *Chlamydia pneumoniae,* herpes virus, and mycoplasma in the causation of atherosclerosis and coronary artery disease.

L-carnitine is a nutrient made within our body from two amino acids, lysine and methionine. This compound is found in high concentration in beef, pork, and bacon. Intestinal bacteria via a series of steps has been shown to convert l-carnitine to a substance , trimethylamine-N-oxide or better known as TMAO. This compound has recently been demonstrated to accelerate

[88] Whether the origin or progression of a fatty plaque has an infectious component (viral or bacterial) is not clear. In a Johns Hopkins study reported in the August 18, 1998 issue of Circulation:626-633, C. pneumoniae infection was linked to the development of atherosclerosis. The team studied coronary artery plaque samples from 60 Alaska Natives who died from non heart disease causes. In 75% of plaque samples, the bacterium was discovered within macrophage foam cells, which are known to be involved in early atherosclerosis. This finding further strengthens the link between C. pneumoniae infection and coronary heart disease.

atherosclerosis in mice. This may be an explanation of why there is a link between high levels of red meat consumption and cardiovascular risk. Teens who take carnitine as a dietary supplement should be made aware of this connection. This is one more reason to be wary of dietary supplements.

PRODUCT/100 grams	CARNITINE
Beef steak	**95 mg**
Ground beef	**94 mg**
Pork	**27.7 mg**
Bacon	**23.3 mg**
Tempeh	**19.5 mg**
Cod fish	**5.6 mg**
Chicken breast	**3.9 mg**
American cheese	**3.7 mg**
Cottage cheese	**1.1 mg**

A recent study from the Cleveland Clinic[89] found that, "increased blood carnitine levels in patients strongly predicted increased risks for cardiovascular disease and major adverse events such as heart attack, stroke and death," but his was only true, "in subjects who also had high TMAO levels."

THE MEDITERRANIAN DIET

Ancel Keys noticed that heart disease varied tremendously throughout the world. Finland had extremely high rates while Japanese remained low until they moved to the United States and adopted a Western Diet. Those with the lowest rates of heart disease were from Crete. They ate quite a bit of fat, but mostly unsaturated fats such as those found in fish and olive oil. He promoted the Mediterranean diet. It was not a "no fat" diet. Dr. Keys recommended a diet of about 30% fat. It was one of substituting

[89] Nature Med. 2013. Doi:10. 1038/nm.3145.

fats from highly saturated fat diet to one that was mostly monounsaturated and high in omega-3 essential fatty acids.

A recent study of the Mediterranean diet was published in the New England Journal of Medicine (NEJM 2/25/2013). In this trial that took place in Spain, researchers randomly assigned study volunteers **at risk** of heart disease to a Mediterranean or standard low-fat diet for five years, allowing the team to single out the effect of diet. Almost 7500 older adults with diabetes or other heart **risks** were divided into one of three groups. Subjects continued the medications they had, such as statins or diabetic drugs. Two groups were instructed to eat a Mediterranean diet-one supplemented with extra-virgin olive oil and the other with nuts. The third study group ate a "control" diet, which emphasized low-fat dairy products, grains, fruits and vegetables. Over the next five years, 288 study participants had a heart attack, stroke or died of any type of cardiovascular disease. People on both Mediterranean diets were 28-30% less likely to develop cardiovascular disease than those on the general low-fat diet. This is the first randomized trial of any diet pattern to show benefit among people at risk, but initially without heart disease.

Critics of this trial state that the benefits were overstated. Repeated studies need to be done to confirm these results.

The Diet: It is a blend of Mediterranean diet components-not one particular ingredient-that promotes heart health.

a. Legumes, fresh vegetables, fruits as desserts and cooking with olive oil.
b. Fresh seafood and fish
c. Discouraging refined breads, pasta, and sweets, sodas, red meats and processed meats (salami, bologna, pepperoni, jerky)
d. Replacing a high-carbohydrate or high saturated fat snacks with a handful of nuts

e. Water or for those adults, red wine with meals, instead of hard alcohol.

Although this was a high risk group, I see no reason that children should wait until they become high risk!

Ancel Keys died at the age of 101. His wife died when she was 97.

LOW FAT DIETS

In the 1960's-1970's heart disease was still believed to be caused primarily by stress. Nathan Pritikin popularized his extremely low fat, high complex carbohydrate diet with claims that this diet could reverse the atherosclerotic plaque and reverse the symptoms of type 2 diabetes mellitus. Pritikin suggested we eat whole, unprocessed, and natural carbohydrate-rich foods, such as grains, and vegetables. Preferred foods included:

Brown rice, millet, barley, oats, dark green, leafy vegetables, onions, potatoes, squash, beans (black turtle beans, chickpeas, , lentils, and pinto beans), apples, pears, strawberries and bananas.

Some processed whole-grain foods, such as oatmeal are on the plan. White flour pasta is permitted as long as it is with vegetables.

Other guidelines:

Small portions of lean beef, chicken, and low-fat dairy products.

Fish: three servings per week of salmon or other fish rich in omega-3 fatty acids. Avoidance of any fried foods, dressing with fat, and fatty sauces. Eat three meals a day plus two snacks. Stay

active and avoid salty foods. Artificial sweeteners are OK on the plan.[90]

He published his "Live Longer Now" that rationally explained, step-by-step, his interpretation of how the atheroma developed within arterial walls. His nutrition program along with mild daily exercise, demonstrated the arrest of further development of arterial disease.

His hypothesis was rejected by the mainstream medical establishment.

As a pediatric resident I was taught that hypertension, adult onset diabetes, and heart disease were the inevitable consequences of aging. They were to be treated with medications! The idea that these diseases were due to a high fat diet stoked my interest in nutrition.

Dr. Dean Ornish's low fat diet is also based on vegetables, grains, and fruits. His reduced stress program for reversing heart disease is another major component and in many ways similar to the Pritikin Principle. It is a respected University of California based program.

THE CHINA STUDY by T. Colin Campell, PhD is mentioned here because this is the diet recently followed by former President Bill Clinton. It is a plant-based diet that excludes meats, eggs, poultry and all dairy. Dr. Campell recommends eating

[90] You may be turning to sugar substitutes and artificial sweeteners to avoid sucrose, fructose, HFCS, or calories. They are widely used in processed foods, including baked goods soft drinks, powdered drink mixes, candy, puddings, canned foods, jams and jellies, dairy products, and many other foods and beverages.

The safety of artificial sweeteners continues to be debated. There are concerns over aspartame's Nutrasweet & Equal) and sucralose (Splenda) safety, but according to the Mayo Clinic report on artificial sweeteners (see MayoClinic.com), the National Cancer Institute, and other health agencies, there's no sound scientific evidence that any of the artificial sweeteners approved for use in the US, cause cancer or other serious health problems. There have been no long term studies.

whole foods and that one should not be relying on the idea that nutrient supplementation is the way to go.

The president lives primarily on beans and other legumes, vegetables and fruit, although he will, on rare occasions, eat fish.

THE INFLAMATION HYPOTHESIS

The hypothesis that inflammation is a core contributor to the development of heart disease and stroke is gaining more support as studies are showing this to be another major risk factor.

Inflammation may cause an atheroma (plaque) within the wall of an artery to explosively rupture through the artery wall. The body reacts by forming a blood clot and when this clot obstructs a heart artery, a heart attack is triggered. A plaque causing clot from a diseased brain artery can travel to the brain causing a stroke.

C-Reactive Protein (CPR) is elevated in patients before, during and after a heart attack or stroke. It has been observed that markers of inflammation such as an elevated C-Reactive Protein seems to be a predictor of future heart attack and is now routinely measured in adult patients.

Researchers continue to search for foods that promote inflammation, such as fatty acids, and microorganisms that might be triggers of acute heart attack via the inflammatory pathway. Influenza is a viral disease that is often underestimated. It is more than a slight "cold" and many heart attacks are followed by this illness due to the body's inflammatory response to viruses and bacteria. "Free Radicals" are also suspected of causing inflammation and damage to the cellular lining of blood vessels. To prevent free radical damage, the body has a defense system of anti-oxidants. Anti-oxidants are molecules that can safely interact with free radicals and terminate the chain reaction before the arterial lining cells are damaged. The body can't manufacture the required vitamin antioxidants, such as vitamin

C, beta-carotene, vitamin E and lycopene. These must come from the diet (not pills!). Foods, such as blueberries, raspberries, blackberries, strawberries and cranberries are excellent sources of antioxidants.

The **Zone Diet** popularized by Dr. Barry Seals, aims to reduce cellular inflammation. To reach proper hormone balance he suggests fat consumption is essential for "burning" fat. He claims that the relatively high proportion of carbohydrate in low-fat/ high carbohydrate diets, compared with protein, increases the production of insulin, causing the body to store fat. When insulin levels are neither too high or too low, then specific anti-inflammatory chemicals called eicosanoids, are released. Sears claims that a 30:40 ratio of protein to carbohydrate triggers this effect. He calls this ,"the ZONE." Sears says that these natural anti-inflammatories are heart and health-friendly. No direct studies to verify his conclusions have been performed.

"Health Food" stores promote all type of antioxidants as beverages or in pill form to their clients as nutritional supplements over-stating their power to prevent heart attacks. Many of these clients thus continue their lethal dietary habit of consuming a high saturated fat, high simple sugars, highly refined foods, fried foods, and high salt foods.

THE SUGAR HYPOTHESIS

Sugar as a cause of cardiovascular disease, was reported by Dr. John Yudkin in Lancet, a respected British medical journal, in 1964. Yudkin studied levels of dietary sucrose in patients with coronary atherosclerotic disease. He claimed that dietary sugar might be involved causally in coronary heart disease and type 2 diabetes. In another study that followed, it was shown that the

sugar intake of men with heart attacks or artery disease was twice that of others without cardiovascular disease. Studies he conducted on sugar indicated that they raised blood triglycerides and insulin levels. Dr. Yudkin was an early advocate of low carbohydrate diets later to be popularized by Dr. Robert Atkins, a cardiologist, and modified in the South Beach Diet. Most are designed to appeal to those who wish to loose weight and get a smaller gut.

Dr. Yudkin's claims were pushed aside when subsequent studies did not confirm the original claims that sucrose was a major contributor to coronary heart disease risk.

Once again, investigators and endocrinologists are claiming simple sugars, especially sucrose, fructose and high fructose corn syrup (HFCS) to be the culprits involved in our epidemic of obesity, diabetes type 2, and cardiovascular disease.(The Metabolic Syndrome). They argue that a high protein, low simple carbohydrate diet offers multiple benefits to health.

In 1972 Dr.Yudkin's book, "Pure,White and Deadly" was published by Davis-Poynter Ltd. and " Sweet and Dangerous" was published in 1972 by Bantam Books.

THE PALEOLITHIC DIET

Paleolithic nutrition refers to a "hunter gatherer" diet, first published by Walter L.Voegtlin in 1975 as the Stone Age Diet: Based on in-depth Studies of Human Ecology and the Diet of Man. His thesis was that humans are carnivorous animals and our ancestor's diet was carnivorous-chiefly fats and protein with only small amounts of carbohydrates.

This diet has its roots in evolutionary biology. The charge is that our biochemistry and physiology are tuned to life conditions that existed some 10,000 years ago and that our bodies are genetically virtually the same as they were at the end o the

Paleolithic Era some 20,000 years ago. Proponents of this diet say that excessive consumption of the Western Diet and sedentary life style contribute to many of the so-called diseases of civilization. There are no large or well controlled studies to support this diet.

Which diet (by diet I mean healthy, nutritious meals) is best? The Atkins meat based high fat plan, The Yudkin's very low sugar diet, the Pritikin plant based low fat plan or the low inflammatory diets? Or is it the Paleolithic Diet. Read on before you decide.

The above mentioned diets are either "weight loss" diets or diets designed to treat those who are sick, with heart disease, diabetes, gout, arthritis, metabolic syndrome, and the endless illnesses blamed on "old age."

Personally, I favor the Mediterranean Diet for children and adults. Do not confuse this with a high pasta and cheese diet. Olive oil is my favorite for cooking along with canola oil for baking. Although some olive oil enthusiasts suggest using a small amount of olive oil as a supplemental beverage, I do not. They belong to the, "more is better" school. The key is fresh vegetables, legumes, whole grains, nuts, poultry, fish, eggs, small amounts of very lean meats, and whole grains. Added sugar or juice and especially sugar-fat food combinations (as found in most "fast foods") should be avoided as a regular visitor.

The Mediterranean "Diet" is not for losing weight. It is a diet for healthy living and designed to prevent many of the infirmities that blight The Golden Years.

FIBER

▲ ▲ ▲

What grandmother referred to as "roughage" is now called fiber. Until recently it was believed that fiber was of no nutritional value. In fact, food processors removed the fiber from grains such as wheat and rice to "improve" textures and color. They called this refining, which gave flour the smooth white color and texture for our cakes, breads and cereals.

Bran is often used synonymously, but incorrectly, with the term dietary fiber. Dietary fiber is that part of cereal grains and all vegetables not digested and absorbed by the intestines. Fiber can be divided into two broad categories, soluble (as found in oat bran, barley, beans, carrots, peas, sweet potatoes, yams, figs, berries, and fruit pectin such as apples and grapefruit,) and insoluble (as found in wheat bran, corn, black-eyed peas, figs and berries). Most plants contain both types in varying amounts, but certain foods are particularly rich in one or the other. Whole grains are quite complex and contain substances we know little about nutritionally. Besides minerals such as selenium, copper, magnesium, vitamin E, phytic and phenolic acids, there are lignins, phytoestrogens (plant estrogens) antioxidants, and other unknown factors. The best way to get fiber plus these other nutrient is to eat a diet rich in complex carbohydrates. Seeds and nuts are also excellent sources, but they should be eaten very sparingly because of their high fat content.

Now we know that in addition to preventing constipation, insoluble fiber may inhibit the development of colon and rectal cancer[91], reduce the likelihood of gallstones and decrease the risk of diverticulosis.

Diverticulosis is a condition in which tiny pouches, called diverticula, form within the wall of the colon. When the pouches trap food, they may become painfully inflamed (diverticulitis) causing pain, bleeding, flatulence, diarrhea or constipation. Experts estimate that in North America, a third of people over 45 and two-thirds of those over 85 have it. By reducing constipation, the insoluble dietary fiber may help to prevent the development of diverticula and relieve the inflammation once it occurs. Soluble fiber improves blood sugar in adult onset diabetes and type I diabetes by slowing the absorption of sugar in the intestines, thus reducing the need for more insulin. Soluble fiber also reduces blood cholesterol by lowering LDL ("bad cholesterol").

What isn't clear is whether it's the fiber alone that causes the benefits attributed to fiber. Those adults who consumes 25-30 grams of fiber a day, in study after study have reduced the risk of cancer, heart attacks, diabetes, and the symptoms of diverticulosis. **It is assumed that this is because of the fiber** in the diet, but it may be the fiber **plus the ingredients found in high fiber foods** (grains, vegetables and fruit). Isolating a single ingredient, like fiber or beta carotene and giving it as a supplement, in the form of a capsule, has yielded disappointing results. There is

[91] A diet rich in fiber may not protect you from colon cancer. The health and eating habit of 88,000 women were studied by Charles Fuchs and colleagues at Harvard University for over a 16 years. In contrast to some previous findings, they determined that women who consumed at least 25 grams of fiber a day were just as likely to get colon or rectal cancer as women who ate half that amount. More research is needed to settle this issue, but this study illustrates how important it is to keep an open mind and continue to restudy (research) accepted "truths." Nevertheless, fiber should remain an important part of our daily diet.

something about eating whole foods in the form of whole grains, fruits and vegetables that scientists have not unraveled. That is one reason why I do not encourage the fad of sprinkling bran over your food. In fact, one of the more common causes of recurrent belly pain in childhood is caused by bran (bran-bellyache).

Look for cereals that are whole grain and high in fiber. Avoid the sugar-added cereals. This may be difficult to tell since in the Nutrition Facts label sugar is not listed as "sugar added" but only Total Sugar. This sugar may be only from the fruit, such as raisins. Avoid the food when HFCS (High Fructose Corn Syrup) is on the Ingredient List.

Although there is no RDA for fiber, the recommended intake is 0.2 grams of dietary fiber per pound to a maximum of 35 grams daily. To calculate the recommended dietary fiber for a 25 pound child: (25 X 0.2 = 5 grams of dietary fiber). For a 50 pound child, it would be 50 X 0.2 = 10 grams of dietary fiber. Or for a more rapid calculation: for every 25 pounds of body weight, 5 grams of fiber is recommended. Thus a 75 pound child's recommended dietary fiber intake is 15 grams.

EXAMPLES OF CEREALS HIGH IN WHOLE GRAIN AND LOW IN SUGAR[92]

COLD CEREALS	HOT CEREALS
Kashi Heart to Heart	
Uncle Sam original	
Roman Meal Multi Grain	
Kashi Go Lean	Steel Cut Irish Oatmeal
Kellogg's Almond Raisin Muslix	Wheatena
Raisin Bran Extra Grain	Erewhon Brown Rice Cream

[92] One easy way to select a dry cereal for your children is to have them choose a cereal they like as long as it has at least 3 grams of fiber. Most cereals that have three or more grams of fiber are nutritious.

Kellogg's All-Bran, Ban Flakes
Kellogg's Mini-Wheats
Post Bran Flakes
Barbara's Shredded Wheat
Cheerios
Kellogg's Mini-Wheats
General Mills Cheerios
Post Shredded Wheat Original
Kellogg Unfrosted Mini-Wheats Bite Size
Arrowhead Mills Oat Bran
Kashi Breakfast Pilaf

INSTANT HOT CEREALS

Quaker Instant Oatmeal-regular
Arrowhead Mills Instant Multigrain Cereal
Mother's Instant Oatmeal
Roman Meal Instant Cream of Rye

For granola lovers, choose the low-fat granola cereals such as Bear Naked Granola.

The practical side of finding suitable high fiber foods may be confusing unless you buy unprepared foods. For example, the label on bread may show a reasonable amount of fiber, but it may have been added from peas or other foods. This fiber may prevent constipation and diverticulosis, but it doesn't have all the ingredients of antioxidants and phytochemicals found in whole grain. A manufacturer may add inulin fiber to cereal to get a healthy looking label. Inulin rapidly traverses the gut and bacteria in the large intestine love this material and convert it into fatty acid and lots of gas. The result is much unwelcome flatulence and bloating.

The fiber in a product should come from the whole food and not as added fiber.

Here are some hints to help you break through the utter confusion set before the average and even sophisticated consumer.

<u>If the label says:</u>

Whole grain or whole wheat - <u>it's a whole grain.</u>

<u>If the label says:</u>

Cracked wheat, "made with whole grain," "made with whole wheat," multi-grain, oat bran, oatmeal, pumpernickel, seven-grain, seven-bran, nine-grain, etc., stoned wheat, wheat, wheat-berry, whole bran - <u>it's mostly refined grain!</u>

*All serving sizes are for cooked vegetables

EXAMPLES OF HIGH FIBER LOW CALORIE FOODS[93]

Food	Serving size	Fiber (grams)	Calories
Figs	**3**	**3.6**	**190**
Dried Figs	**3**	**3.6**	**190**
Apple[94]	**1**	**3.5**	**81**
Pear	**1/2 (large)**	**3.1**	**61**
Carrots	**2/3 cup**	**3.1**	**32**
Strawberries	**1 cup**	**3.0**	**45**
Broccoli	**2/3 cup**	**2.9**	**26**
Spinach	**2/3 cup**	**2.8**	**28**
Orange	**1**	**2.6**	**62**
Zucchini	**2/3 cup**	**2.4**	**15**
Prunes	**2**	**2.0**	**40**
Blueberries	**1/2 cup**	**2.0**	**39**
Peach[95]	**1**	**1.9**	**37**

Juicers[96] are very popular and may be fine as long as you use a juicer that doesn't discard the fiber pulp. There are juicers

[93] J. Am. Diet. Assoc. 86: 732, 1986

[94] All serving sizes are for cooked vegetables

[95] With skin

[96] Vita-Mixer (often promoted in Costco Wholesale)

that use all the fruit or vegetable. Remember, these juicers or blenders slice the food rapidly and finely. This increases the surface area of the food and permits it to be digested and absorbed more rapidly. Satiety is delayed and as a result more blended food is swallowed along with many more calories.

Although this is a good way to introduce vegetables to the picky eater, it can quickly add enormous amounts of calories to the already overweight child or teen.

EXAMPLES OF WORST FOODS

By pointing out these foods, I do not wish to be telling you what to eat or feed your child. My goal is to give you the tools of understanding the importance of limiting sodium, sugar, saturated fat and highly refined foods in your diet in order to avoid obesity, heart disease, diabetes, and many diseases once believed to be the inevitable consequences of aging. It is easier to prevent these diseases than to reverse them.

Let me remind you of a couple of the worst foods that are especially attractive to teens and young adults:

1. Anything made with Alfredo sauce, a sauce for pasta incorporating butter, cream, garlic, and Parmesan cheese.

2. Carbonara sauce is another pasta sauce made with bacon or ham, eggs, and cream. Typical nutrition facts-1440 calories; 88grams fat, that is equivalent to 6 doughnuts! And 3000mg of sodium.

3. Deep dish Pizza with sausage contains about 2300 calories, with 164 grams of fat and a whopping 4900 mg of sodium.

4. Chicken or turkey pot pie. Check the Nutrition Facts Label and see whether or not you agree.

VITAMINS

▲ ▲ ▲

Vitamins are organic compounds that **cannot by synthesized by our bodies** and are necessary in **minute quantities** in our diet to keep the body in good condition.

If our bodies were maintained by a diet containing only purified proteins, carbohydrates, fats and the necessary minerals, it would not be possible to sustain life. Vitamins are necessary as an accessory food factor. They act as **biocatalysts** within the body. That is, they promote necessary chemical reactions in the body, without being consumed in the reactions. They function as **co-enzymes** or parts of co-enzymes. For the vitamin to work it must first enter a cell in the body and combine with a particular kind of protein called an apoenzyme. When a co-enzyme attaches to an apoenzyme, a complete or holoenzyme is formed. Extremely small amounts of vitamins are needed. Once all the apoenzymes in the body are saturated to form complete enzymes, more vitamins will collect in the body fluids and be stored, or the excess will be excreted. The vitamins are generally divided into two major groups: fat-soluble and water-soluble. Fat-soluble vitamins are usually found associated with the lipids (fats) of natural foods. These include Vitamins A, D, E, and K. The water-soluble group includes Vitamin C and the vitamins of the B complex.

The RDA for a vitamin is enough to saturate our entire body with that vitamin. Unlike water-soluble vitamins[97], the fat-soluble vitamins are stored in our body fat and can be toxic if large amounts build up. So again, we are reminded that too much of a good thing can be harmful. Or, if not harmful, then wasteful since in a normal person most of the water soluble vitamin supplements wind up in the toilet.

Many diseases of mankind, including beriberi, scurvy, night blindness, and pellagra, are known to be caused by lack of these essential food factors. These vitamins were originally assigned letters of the alphabet. Now that we have been able to identify the chemical structures of vitamins, nutritionists prefer to use their chemical names rather than the letters. In some cases the letters formerly assigned to the vitamins have been dropped entirely. Biotin has been substituted for Vitamin H. Folic acid has been substituted for Vitamin M.

[97] Recent research has demonstrated that, while water-soluble vitamins from food cannot generally reach dangerous levels, supplements should still be used with caution. The latest recommendations from the National Academy of Sciences (NAS), for example, call for 1.3 to 1.7 milligrams of vitamin B-6. Although some people claim a very high intake of vitamin B-6 can produce valuable health benefits, doses greater than 100 milligrams have caused nerve damage and are listed as a health risk in the new NAS recommendations. The report also warns of toxic effects from excessive doses of niacin.

WATER SOLUBLE

Vitamin levels for the water-soluble vitamins are measured in either milligrams (mg., thousandths of a gram) or micrograms (mcg., thousandths of a milligram).
The vitamins of the B complex and their synonyms are listed with the accepted current name first and the historical names in parenthesis.

1. Thiamin (Vitamin B-1, antiberiberi substance, antineuritic vitamin, aneurine)

2. Riboflavin (Vitamin B-2, lactoflavin)

3. Niacin (Vitamin B-3, P-P factor of Goldberger, nicotinic acid)

4. Pyridoxine (Vitamin B-6, rat antidermatitis factor)

5. Pantothenic acid (Vitamin B-5, filtrate factor, chick antidermatitis factor)

6. Lipoic acid (thioctic acid, acetate replacement factor)[98]

7. Biotin (Vitamin H, anti-egg white injury factor)

8. Folate (liver lactobacillus casei factor, Vitamin M, fermentation residue factor, pteroylglutamic acid, folic acid group)

9. Inositol (mouse anti-alopecia factor)

10. Para-aminobenzoic acid; PABA

11. Vitamin B-12 (cyanocobalamin, cobalmin, antipernicious anemia factor, extrinsic factor of Castle)

[98] These members of the B complex are not considered to be vitamins in humans.

PABA

WATER SOLUBLE

Ascorbic Acid (Vitamin C)
B Complex group

FAT SOLUBLE

Vitamin levels for the fat-soluble nutrients A, D, E, and K are measured in international units (IUs).
Vitamin A (retinol)
Vitamin D (calciferol)
Vitamin E (tocopherol)
Vitamin K

Vitamins act both independently and often together. Most vitamin deficiency disease is seen predominantly in areas of the world where war and famine exist, and the cases usually show mixed deficiency. It is more common for isolated deficiency to occur in specific circumstances, for example: Vitamin K deficiency as an isolated event occurs in infancy. The infant most vulnerable is the breastfed

newborn. Normal adults rarely lack Vitamin K. In the newborn, however, the quantity of the vitamin derived from the mother is small. At birth the intestines do not contain the bacteria necessary to manufacture vitamin K and the breast milk does not supply it. Mild Vitamin K deficiency in the newborn is common. Very low levels, as a result of the deficiency, may cause hemorrhages in the newborn. This disaster can easily be prevented by giving the infant oral or intramuscular Vitamin K once soon after birth.

Another situation is found in Vitamin D, the "sunshine vitamin" deficiency. There is a saying in the Alps of Austria, "Fall baby - spring rickets!" Austrian winters are long and cold. Infants are wrapped and away from sunlight from October until late March. The result is that eight months after birth the infant has soft bones and the extreme irritability which mark rickets. Most of the infants who become deficient are fed cow's milk which has no Vitamin D. Human breast milk is also deficient in Vitamin D, but the illness is more rare in breast fed infants. Strangely, the deficiency is also seen in the Caribbean where it is common practice in some cultures to wrap infants completely to keep them protected from the sun.

Vitamin deficiency is very rare in the USA because fresh vegetables are readily available year round. In addition, bread, flour, cornmeal, corn grits, macaroni, and spaghetti products as well as infant cereals and dry cereals are vitamin enriched. In spite of this, there remains a vulnerable group that still exists in this country.

At risk is the person on a high level macrobiotic diet whose diet is not varied but is mostly rice. Beware of bizarre fad diets, regardless of how eloquently they are presented.

Another at risk group, is the elderly bachelor or widower who may prepare his own foods. Both are particularly prone to the development of Vitamin C deficiency, a syndrome termed "bachelor scurvy." They're not eating enough fruit. Food faddists who avoid raw foods, particularly fruits and vegetables, are at risk to develop Vitamin C deficiencies. Deficiency malnutrition is common among alcoholics, the poor, the elderly, and the chronically ill. In contrast, vitamin excess is a disorder of the well-to-do.

A megavitamin is a vitamin given in a dose ten times the RDA or more. If there is a specific defect in a person's body chemistry limiting absorption of a vitamin or preventing normal amounts of vitamins from getting across cell walls into the body tissues, then megadose vitamins may be extremely helpful. There are, for example, infants born with defective apoenzymes or inborn errors of metabolism. By giving such a patient megadoses of a vitamin you can force the co-enzyme (vitamin) reaction by mass action. Vitamin D resistant rickets is one example where mega-vitamins can be used to good advantage. Folate or folic acid[99] as a 1mg to 10mg (1000 micrograms to 10,000 micrograms) daily megadose supplementation before pregnancy may prevent certain types of cleft lips and palates and is currently under investigation.

Claims that niacin regulates blood sugar and is useful in the "megavitamin" treatment of schizophrenia or that it is of value in the prevention of heart problems have not been substantiated by adequate controlled studies. Instead, what we have mostly are testimonials by people, including physicians, that they "felt better" after taking megadoses of these vitamins. It is important to keep in mind that these feeling are based far more on faith and wishful thinking than on scientific fact. The same is true for megadose therapy of vitamins and minerals to correct mental retardation or autism. When faced with a situation believed to be "hopeless" most of us are tempted to try anything as long as it is not harmful. The usual feeling is, "What do I have to lose, anyway?" In such a case the decision must remain a personal

[99] Folate or folacin is the natural form of the water-soluble B vitamin found in food. Folic acid is the synthetic form of the vitamin and is found in multivitamins, folic acid supplements, and foods fortified with folic acid. Folate is 30%-50% less bioavailable than folic acid. This is because folate is a "polyglutamate" and the body must convert it to a "monoglutamate" before it can be absorbed. Folic acid, the synthetic form of the vitamin, is a "monoglutamate" and requires no conversion for absorption. This information is of practical value because to obtain the recommended daily 400 micrograms of folic acid from foods, an individual must consume about 800 micrograms of natural folate. It may be very difficult to obtain the needed amount of folate from the diet alone since a considerable amount of folate may be destroyed when foods are cooked, processed, or stored. Women considering pregnancy should begin taking a daily folic acid supplement at least three months before and continue taking it for the entire pregnancy. Many public health advisors suggest that all women of child bearing age should begin taking daily folic acid supplements and continue until menopause. These authorities remind us that at least 50% of all pregnancies in the USA are unplanned. See page ****** for more information on folate and prevention of birth deformities such as neural tube defects, cleft lip and palate, and early miscarriage.

one. But be careful. Some of these concoctions are not without danger. Hope should never be taken away from anyone in a desperate situation, but false hope can only lead to disillusionment. When someone realizes he has been "used" or "taken" by a professional opportunist during a vulnerable moment in his or her life, it magnifies the feelings of sorrow and loss.

Consumers are receiving an unprecedented flood of information, some of which is properly analyzed while some is widely publicized without proper scrutiny. This often misguided nutritional information is actively promoted by "health food stores" and by doctors who practice unconventional or "fringe" medicine. The Internet is loaded with these "nutritional" promotions. Caveat emptor-buyer beware!

The idea that "natural" vitamins provide special benefits for our bodies has been promoted by manufacturers and retailers of these vitamins. Vitamins have the same properties whether natural or synthetic. Many vitamins labeled natural or organic are not what you might imagine those terms to mean. Rose hips Vitamin C tablets are made from natural rose hips, which have natural vitamin C combined with chemical ascorbic acid, the same Vitamin C used in standard tablets. If no vitamin C were added to the tablet " it would have to be as big as a golf ball." Makers of "natural" vitamin C often suggest that synthetic vitamins do not contain other hidden or not well-known micro nutrients that are included in the natural forms. They point to the "associated factors," flavonoids, proto-pectins and minerals of the whole fruit, including the so-called "P" factors. Although the rational conclusion is to eat the entire fruit or vegetable to obtain all the nutritional value, instead the consumer is told their diet needs a promoted supplement. Natural B complex vitamins are mostly synthetic chemicals added to yeast and other bases. Vitamin E[100] products are derived from vegetable oils, but in order to concentrate the vitamin in a capsule, various chemical solvents must be used. The vegetable material is grown with the usual pesticides

[100] See section on Vitamin E for more information on this vitamin.

and chemical fertilizers. Finally, the gelatin capsule must contain a preservative so that it won't turn rancid. Since the vitamins are identical, no one can tell them apart, neither in a test tube nor in an animal. The health food industry designs its advertisements to make you feel vulnerable plus inadequate so you have a need to play it safe and purchase the magical nutrient. How far have we come since Ponce de Leon marched through Florida seeking the "Fountain of Youth?"

See section on Vitamin E for more information on this vitamin.

The following information on selected vitamins is provided because there is currently special interest in these nutrients. For more in depth information on the vitamins I have omitted, visit your local bookstore, public library or Internet and refer to the most current texts.

VITAMIN C (ASCORBIC ACID)

Vitamin C is needed daily in the diet because our bodies cannot manufacture or store it. An adequate supply of vitamin C prevents scurvy. Scurvy is a disease found in persons with little or no vitamin C intake over a prolonged period. In scurvy there is bruising, infected gums with loose teeth, bleeding into the joints and muscles of the legs and arms. Finally, if not corrected, jaundice develops, edema (swelling), fever, convulsions and finally death. This is the classic description of scurvy, and in all my years of practice, I have never seen a case in a child. So please do not think your bruises are due to vitamin C deficiency.

Cigarette smoking and birth control pills increase the need for vitamin C. No case has yet been reported of any individual who ate one fruit or vegetable daily and developed scurvy because of smoking. Megadoses of vitamin C have been used to treat viral illnesses such as the common cold, hepatitis, influenza, infectious mononucleosis, and pneumonia. The most common side effects of such treatment have been stomach and intestinal upset, diarrhea, abdominal cramping, and flatulence. Lowering the dose of vitamin C usually eliminates these symptoms. The proponents of this type of vitamin therapy suggest that the dose should be increased to the amount needed to produce these symptoms, then the dose should be lowered slightly. Although there is no strong evidence that vitamin C prevents the "common cold," there is some evidence that it may decrease the symptoms and shorten the duration of the illness. Many of my patients take vitamin C supplements and I see as many of these patients for illness as I see who do not take vitamin C. This, of course, is a non-controlled observation! Of greater importance is the value of vitamin C in preventing the conversion of dietary nitrates into a potent carcinogen, nitrosamine. Vitamin C taken daily as a supplement, or even better, daily consumption of foods high in vitamin C, could decrease the risk of intestinal cancer by preventing nitrosamine formation. Vitamin C also blocks the bacteria Hilocobacter pylori, a major cause of stomach ulcer and, possibly, stomach cancer. Citrus fruits[101], strawberries, melons, tomatoes, broccoli, spinach, potatoes, green and red peppers, are all good sources of vitamin C, as are a number of tropical fruits, such as kiwi and papaya. At this time there is a flurry of interest in Vitamin C by eye specialist because according to animal studies, high levels of vitamin C in the eye appear to protect against the cataract-inducing effects of ultraviolet radiation from the sun. Prolonged exposure to ultraviolet light is believed to contribute to cataract formation. Middle aged people who took vitamin C supplements for many years lowered their risk of cataracts by as much as 80%.

[101] The citrate in orange juice inhibits the formation of calcium stones in the kidney.

Fortunately, most of the warnings about possible toxicity of vitamin C when it is used as a drug are exaggerated. Compared with the drugs we use daily in medical practice, "over the counter" or socially, vitamin C is a remarkably safe substance.

The story behind discovering the cause of scurvy is fascinating. During the 18th and 19th century Great Britain needed a large navy to protect and service its colonial based economy. Scurvy became prevalent when sailors began to spend months at sea without fresh fruit or vegetables. It was of economic importance for Britain to find out what caused scurvy. In 1795, lime juice was given to all British sailors on the recommendation of the Scottish physician, James Lund, who knew that the Dutch had given citrus fruit to its sailors for several hundred years. Gradually, scurvy began to disappear from British sailing ships. That is why British sailors became known as "Limeys."

When I was a student I was told by one of my professors that the American naval medical community refused to believe the claim that limes prevented scurvy. To test the theory, so the story goes, Florida key limes where collected and given to American sailors who were at sea for months. The key limes did not protect the American sailors from scurvy, therefore the theory was rejected. We now know that Florida key limes are the only citrus not to contain vitamin C! It took many more years before citrus fruit was introduced to the American navy.

VITAMIN A
(RETINOL OR BETA-CAROTENE)

As a child, the worst part of my day was preparing for bed. That was the time for **Cod Liver Oil.** In those years water soluble vitamins had not been made thus the natural vitamin A was given to most children of my generation. The oil was so horrific, I can still taste and smell these vitamin drops. This experience must have been shared by other children because one major complication of giving cod liver oil was pneumonia. Small amounts of the oil would get into the lungs after a struggling child had a gagging or choking spell. This fat soluble vitamin, found in its natural state, was so irritating to lung tissue that a severe chemical pneumonia developed when the vitamin drops were not totally swallowed but accidentally went down "the wrong tube." Fortunately, we now have a water soluble form and that's what's in children's poly-vitamin drops.

Vitamin A is found in animal products such as liver oils, liver, and egg yolk. Retinol is another name for it because it is needed for proper vision. Beta carotene[102] is a provitamin and the body can convert it to vitamin A in the liver. A provitamin, or precursor, is a substance the body can make into a vitamin. It is the carotene that makes vegetables yellow. It is also in green vegetables, but the dark green chlorophyll color conceals it. About 90% of the storable vitamin A is in the liver. People with diabetes, low thyroid hormone and those who use a lot of polyunsaturated fatty acids without antioxidants (vitamin E) have a decreased ability to convert beta-carotene to vitamin A. One result of too much carotene in the blood is the formation of a yellow-orange skin color which may be seen in those with untreated diabetes or thyroid disease. This vitamin is needed to maintain normal vision in dim light, is involved in bone and tooth enamel growth, wound healing, and promotes

[102] Beta carotene and other members of the carotenoid family are more than vitamin A precursors, that is, substances that are converted into vitamin A in the body. Today we know of more than 500 different carotenoids. Two carotenoids, lutein and zeaxanthin, may protect the eyes against age-related macular degeneration, which afflicts one in three people over age 75. Another carotenoid, lycopene, may help prevent or delay prostate cancer. There are no RDA's for the various carotenoids. Food composition tables currently used by nutritionists lump beta-carotene and its relatives together under the heading vitamin A, making it difficult to identify good sources of particular carotenoids.

healthy skin and mucous membranes. (the linings of organs, such as the lungs, bladder, stomach and intestines.) Vitamin A improves antibody response and other immune processes to help fight off infection and cancer cells. Because of all the beneficial effects of vitamin A, there was overuse of this vitamin to prevent infection, to improve eyesight, and decrease acne. The complications of the, "if a little works, more must be better" theory, side effects of hypervitaminosis A were encountered, such as terrible headache due to brain swelling, bone and joint pain, hair loss, itching, dry skin, tender bones, weakness, fatigue, and most disastrous, birth defects. Therefore, be sure to remain within the RDA for Vitamin A. Too much beta-carotene can lead to orange-yellow colored skin which was epidemic in the 1970's when drinking lots of carrot juice was the fad. Fortunately, "carotenosis," as it is called, is of no real consequence and will clear when there is a reduction in carotene intake. Beta carotene, one of more than 40 carotenoids found in food, is one of the most potent antioxidants. The carotenoids are believed to work in concert with other antioxidants. Although beta carotene vitamin pills are popular, they have not been shown to reduce the risk of cancer or heart disease. This is disappointing news, but no surprise since vegetables and fruits contain so many different chemicals in various combination. Our basic understanding of how foods protect us from cancer and heart disease is fragmentary. You would never guess how little we know by reading the exaggerated claims on products sold in gyms and "health food" stores. There will always be someone trying to sell you food supplements of dubious value in this multi-billion dollar market. Below is a table highlighting good sources of four of the over 40 known carotenoids. This underscores what people are missing when they rely on supplements alone. Get your carotene the old fashioned way. Eat carrots, broccoli, squash, spinach, and green leafy vegetables, cantaloupe and other deep yellow, orange fruit. The deeper the color, the higher the carotenoid content.

SOURCES OF COMMON CAROTENOIDS[103]

	Beta-Carotene (micrograms)	Lutein & Zeaxanthin (micrograms)	Lycopene (micrograms)
1/2 cup cooked broccoli	1,014	1,404	0
1/2 cup Brussels sprouts	374	1,014	0
1 medium raw carrot	5,688	187	0
1/2 pink grapefruit	1,611	0	4,135
1/2 cup cooked kale	3,055	14,235	0
1 medium peach	86	12	0
1 cup raw spinach	2,296	5,712	0
1 medium tomato	640	123	3,813
3/4 cup tomato juice	1,638	0	15,616

VITAMIN E (TOCOPHEROL)

Vitamin E is another favorite nutrient surrounded with a magical aura. It has been promoted as a substance that increases sexual prowess, fertility, and protects against heart attacks. It is also claimed that vitamin E applied to a healing wound will diminish the scar.

Pure Vitamin E was first isolated from wheat germ oil in 1936. Although alpha tocopherol is the active compound most often designated as vitamin E, there are seven other naturally occurring tocopherols. These are designated as (d & l forms) of alpha, beta, gamma, delta, zeta, epsilon, eta, and 8-methyl-tocotrienol. and their biological activity varies greatly.

[103] Tuft University Diet & Nutrition Letter: Vol.14, No.1, March 1996.

Vitamin E functions as an antioxidant and helps protect polyunsaturated fatty acids in cell membranes and elsewhere in the body. Outside the body it prevents rancidity of oil. Because vitamin E prevents a process called peroxidation within cells, it was hoped that megadoses of it would protect cells against the aging process and therefore prolong youth and prevent heart attacks. Clinical trials have not provided evidence that routine use of vitamin E supplements prevents cardiovascular disease or reduces its morbidity (illness) and mortality. Further research is needed to determine whether supplemental vitamin E has any protective value against coronary heart disease.

Because vitamin E protects cell constituents from the damaging effects of free radicals that, if unchecked, might contribute to cancer development, it was hoped that the formation of carcinogenic nitrosamines formed in the stomach from nitrites in foods might protect against cancer by enhancing the immune system. Unfortunately, human trials and surveys that have attempted to associate vitamin E intake with cancer incidence have found that vitamin E is not beneficial in most cases.

Other studies have shown that vitamin E intake or supplementation did not reduce the risk of prostate cancer.

Very preliminary studies suggest that vitamin E may delay the onset of Alzheimer's disease; however, it is too early to tell whether vitamin E is protective. Other investigators must see whether these results can be duplicated. Meanwhile, the answer is to eat foods containing the more complete form of vitamin E. Fruits and vegetables are the best source of antioxidants because they also provide thousands of phytochemicals that enhance the effects of antioxidants. Rich natural sources of vitamin E are whole grains, breads and cereals, soybeans, wheat germ oil, safflower oil, lettuce, and most green leafy vegetables.

Laboratory rat experiments demonstrated a heightened sexual potency from vitamin E, but unfortunately, in humans large doses can reduce sexual organ function.

Vitamin E deficiency occurs rarely and produces few symptoms, while excesses can cause headaches, tiredness, giddiness, inflammation of the mouth, chapped lips, muscle weakness, low blood sugar and bleeding tendency. By antagonizing the action of vitamin A, large doses of vitamin E can also cause blurred vision.

Some of the worst rashes I've seen came from vitamin E oil repeatedly rubbed on scars. The oil is a potent skin sensitizer. Why then do people use vitamin E on scars and claim benefits? The answer is relatively simple. There's nothing that heals better than a newly healing scar! In addition, any oil is soothing. Yet most experiments show that anything placed on or in a wound slows healing. My advice is to use a pure vegetable oil if you enjoy the soothing effect, but avoid Vaseline and vitamin oils unless you wish to invite red, bumpy, and irritated skin.

VITAMIN D (CALCIFEROL)

SAFE GUIDELINES FOR VITAMIN D SUPPLEMENTATION

AGE	RDA (IU)	UPPER LEVEL (IU)
1 to 3 years	**600**	**2,500**
4 to 8 years	**600**	**3000**
9 to 70 years	**600**	**4000**
71 and older	**800**	**4000**

As discussed earlier, Vitamin D is the "sunshine" vitamin. Because vitamin D is needed for the normal calcification of bone and teeth, it is very important in the development of a healthy child. Vitamin D is actually more like a hormone than a vitamin. It is produced in the skin and released into the blood to affect bone and other tissues. If the intake of vitamin D is low or if the child has inadequate sun exposure, even with sufficient dietary calcium and phosphorous, a child or adult will have poor calcification of bone. Menopausal women who take calcium supplements without vitamin D 3 will not receive optimal benefits from taking calcium. Because most milk is fortified with vitamin D, deficiency of this vitamin in children was seldom a problem in this country. Now with sun screen use, fewer children playing outdoors in the sun, and less milk drinking amongst teenagers, we are now finding more mild vitamin D deficiency.

There is evidence from research done on cultured cells (cells isolated from the body and grown in special solutions of nutrients) and in animals with severe vitamin D deficiency that vitamin D (calciferol) is important for activating the immune system. This discovery, many scientists believe, provides much needed information about the immune system and it is believed that vitamin D is an immune modulator. The "Health Food Industry" is making wild claims from this basic research, including vitamin D's ability to stop or control the common cold. Unfortunately, scientific studies sadly found vitamin D to be as helpful against the common cold as a placebo. Vitamin D is helpful in many other ways and you should consider supplementing your diet with it by taking a daily D3 fish oil supplement or consuming more fatty fish such as salmon, herring and mackerel.

In addition low blood levels of vitamin D may contribute to the development of peripheral arterial disease. This is a condition of the blood vessels that leads to narrowing and hardening of the arteries that supply the leg and feet. The narrowing of the blood vessels leads to decreased blood flow and causes recurrent leg and calf pain and cramping.

Overweight children 6-18 years old are often found to be vitamin D deficient. It is not clear whether it is because they spend too much time indoors in front of the TV and computer screen and out of the sun or because their diet is heavy in calories and not heavy in nutrients. The rates of vitamin D deficiency were higher in Latinos and African-Americans. The particularly high prevalence in severely obese and minority children suggest that targeted screening and treatment guidance is needed.

Vitamin D deficiency is also **linked** to a variety of chronic conditions, such as:

- High blood pressure
- Type 1 diabetes
- Multiple sclerosis.
- Cognitive function
- Depression
- Autoimmune disease

Randomized trials are underway to shed more light on vitamin D, but results won't be forthcoming for another couple of years. In the meantime, there is concern that vitamin D deficiency and inadequacy have been overestimated. The present advice is to keep supplementation within the safe guidelines listed above.

FOLIC ACID (FOLATE)

Folic acid deficiency[104] may be one of the most common vitamin deficiencies in this country. The word comes from the

104

Latin *folium,* which means "foliage," because it is found in leafy vegetables such as spinach, kale, broccoli, asparagus, chard, sprouts, and other "greens." Folic acid (folate) is available from fresh, unprocessed foods. Many fruits contain folic acid, such as oranges, cantaloupe, pineapple, banana, and many berries, including strawberries, loganberries, and boysenberries. Because so many parents and children live on a diet high in processed foods, they are at risk for folic acid deficiency. Folic acid (folate) is need to make DNA, and DNA is needed for cell growth and division. When the body is actively producing cells, as in early pregnancy, there is a tremendous need for extra folate. Since folate, a water soluble B-complex vitamin, is not stored well in the body, humans must consume a constant supply through foods or supplements. If deficiency is present in a pregnant woman, cell division of the fetus stops, and if this is at a critical time in the development of a fetus (unborn infant), organ formation may be incomplete. Such deformities, (called **neural tube defects**), can result in spina bifida, in which the spinal cord resides outside the spinal column. Defects of the face, including cleft lip and palate, may also occur. Children with neural tube defects are more likely to have a variant gene[105] that controls the conversion of the amino acid homocysteine to methionine. This mutation may interfere with an intermediate step in the conversion, preventing the overall process from occurring. Researchers have speculated that too much homocysteine prevents the closure of the neural tube, leading to these defects. If the mother consumes adequate amounts of folic acid prior to conception, the conversion of homocysteine to methionine may still proceed, regardless of the child's genetics, and the neural tube may close. Since these problems occur early in pregnancy, it is especially important for all girls and women of childbearing age to consume a diet high in folate. I recommend that anyone of childbearing

[105] Tolarova. M., A .Goldberg et al. A common mutation in the MTHFR gene is a risk factor for nonsyndromic cleft lip and palate anomalies. Am J Hum Genet 1998.63:A.27

age take **at least a 0.8 mgs supplement daily**.[106] Beginning folate after the critical first few weeks of pregnancy will be too late to correct or prevent the possible damage. When you consider that most women are not even aware of being pregnant until they miss a period, you can see how important it is to develop good dietary habits early. A diet rich in complex carbohydrates, in the form of daily fresh vegetables and fruits is needed if you are to have healthy normal children.

[106] Beginning in 1998, the Food and Drug Administration required that any grain product wishing to market itself as enriched be fortified with 140 micrograms of folic acid per 100 grams of food. This is considered by experts to be too low to significantly prevent the birth defects caused by folic acid deficiency. It is estimated that only 25% of women of childbearing age are consuming the recommended 0.4 mg (400 micrograms) of folic acid every day. The new FDA rule will increase the number of women daily consuming 0.4mg to only 28%. A medical prescription is needed for multivitamins containing 1 mg or more of folic acid. Prescriptions of these prenatal vitamins are available from your physician.

MINERALS

▲ ▲ ▲

There are a number of definitions of the word "mineral." In order to understand what mineral means in nutrition, a quick review of some basic chemistry is necessary. Remember that all matter is composed of atoms. There are different types of atoms, such as oxygen, iron, and zinc atoms. These atoms are the basic building blocks of matter. Different types of atoms can combine to form **chemical compounds**. For example, the atoms hydrogen and oxygen are combined to form the chemical compound, <u>water</u>.

Nutritionists use the term "mineral" to refer to the various types of **atoms** needed by the body. A mineral is an atom or an "**element**" (not a compound such as a vitamin), obtained from food, which is essential to health and is needed in small quantities, sometimes in tiny amounts called "trace elements." Ordinarily, minerals are not eaten in pure form but actually are obtained as part of various compounds in our foods. The body can separate minerals from the food compound in which they are found.

Sodium, calcium, magnesium, and phosphorous are examples of minerals or elements needed by the body, while the minerals, copper, zinc, iron, and iodine are examples of trace elements.

There are 15 major elements of nutritional importance and six are required in relatively large amounts. These include calcium, phosphorous, magnesium, potassium, chloride, and sodium. The remaining nine are essential trace elements: iron, zinc, iodine, manganese, selenium, copper, fluoride, chromium, and molybdenum. These "trace" elements have specific metabolic roles in enzyme systems. Enzymes, as you may recall, are large protein molecules. Most metabolic processes of the body depend on the action of these enzymes.

Not all the minerals listed above will be discussed here. Sodium has already been discussed in Part I. Additional information on calcium and iron is included here, but more information is also provided in Part I since these minerals are so important to normal growth and development.

CALCIUM

Calcium is the most abundant element or mineral in the body. Not only is it important for our skeleton and bones, but also for nerve conduction, blood clotting, skeletal and heart muscle contraction, and many other metabolic processes. Calcium metabolism is complicated and is just beginning to be understood. The amount of calcium consumed is only one part of a chemical chain of events which include vitamin D, parathyroid hormones, intestinal absorption, bone mobilization and deposition, urinary excretion, magnesium, phosphates, dietary protein, gravity or weight bearing exercise and other unknown factors.

Concerns about calcium absorption have arisen in regards to a diet high in phosphorous. This has been of some concern to nutritionists because the consumption of high phosphate foods can decrease absorption. Soft drinks, food additives and meats are high in phosphates. The possible adverse effects of a continual high phosphate (and high protein) intake on calcium and bone loss should not be taken lightly. A high salt diet also contributes heavily to calcium loss. A diet high in convenience foods such as canned or dehydrated soups, or ready to eat frozen dinners provides an excessive salt load to children and adults even if the saltshaker is never used. These long term effects may be of greater consequence than a low calcium diet.

The need for calcium varies in our life cycle. Needs increase during times of rapid growth of skeleton and muscles, such as pregnancy, lactation, infancy and especially during adolescence. Not enough calcium in the diet is common in teenage girls on a high soda, candy bar or "sports bar" diet, but in this group there are multiple nutritional factors that need attention and a "calcium supplement" is only small part of the answer. An unbalanced diet that has excessive salt, phosphorous, protein, and insufficient vitamin D (plus little weight bearing exercise) is a major contributor to calcium deficiency and osteoporosis later in life.

Children and young adults who are bedridden begin to lose calcium and continue to do so until exercise and walking are resumed. Although calcium from dairy products is more completely absorbed, supplementary calcium with vitamin D may be substituted in those who are unable to tolerate milk. If you take calcium supplements, take them at night[107] because it helps reduce calcium loss into the urine which occurs during sleep, but beware of taking too high a dose of calcium because the excessive amount may help form kidney stones[108] or cause other

[107] Some nutritionists and experts on osteoporosis disagree with the notion that it's better to take calcium supplements at bedtime or for that matter, at all. They believe that spreading out a calcium supplement during the day leads to more calcium absorption. Whether you favor one approach over the other should not be the major issue. What is important is that 1000mg to 1200mg of calcium from **all** sources, (diet and supplement), be consumed daily by your teenager to prevent osteoporosis later in life.

[108] If you've had a calcium oxalate kidney stone (your doctor would know), then oxalate-rich foods can cause you trouble. It would be prudent to limit

toxic problems. It is safest to first consult a physician before taking calcium supplements. It is best to avoid supplementation if your dietary calcium is what the RDA suggests. Another piece of sound advice is to cut down on salt, soda (phosphates), and excessive protein because they can remove calcium from the body and counteract the effect of any calcium supplement. **Women who cut the amount of salt in half, from the average of 3450 mg (about 20 times the amount the adult body needs!) to 1725 mg of sodium protect their bones as though a 900 mg calcium supplement had been taken.** When you consider that one in two women over the age of 50 will fracture a bone due to osteoporosis, (a brittle bone condition), you can appreciate how much a high salt diet promotes this condition. A cup of broth, V-8 juice, some cheese, and a salad with anchovies and olives contain enough salt to bump you into calcium losing mode.

You may have read that phytates and oxalates in green vegetables make calcium less bioavailable, and this may be true, but as a practical consideration this is rarely an important problem. Beside the usual list of calcium rich foods. There is little difference in calcium absorption among sources of calcium as long as supplements are taken with food. If taken on an empty stomach, calcium citrate seems to be absorbed best. Calcium carbonate, although the least expensive, should be taken with food for maximum absorption.

Cheese provides substantial nourishment at the expense of over 50% of calories from fat, most of which is saturated, as well as an enormous salt content. Vegetarians who avoid red meat often unwittingly substitute large amount of cheese daily. Nutritionally speaking, cream cheese is considered a fat (such as butter) and should not be classified with milk, yogurt and other

your intake of beans, beets, blueberries, celery, chocolate, grapes, nuts, rhubarb, and spinach. It appears very safe to take the 1200 mg RDA of calcium without worrying about kidney stones, as long as you don't take more as a supplement. Limit **supplemental** calcium to 500 mg.

cheeses.[109] To get the same amount of calcium found in an 8 oz. glass of milk, you'd need to eat 13 ounces (more than a cup and a half) of regular cream cheese! Do not over-consume cheese or dairy products.

RECOMMENDED DAILY ALLOWANCE FOR CALCIUM

Infants	**0 to 6 months**	**210 mg**
	7 months to one year	**270 mg**
Children	**1 to 3**	**700 mg**
	4 to 8	**1000 mg**
Women	**9 to 18**	**1300 mg**
	19 to 50	**1000 mg**
	Over 51	**1200 mg**
Pregnancy and Lactation		**1200 mg**
	Under 19	**1300 mg**
	Over 19	**1000 mg**
Men	**9 to 18**	**1300 mg**
	19 to 50	**1000 mg**
	Over 51	**1200 mg**

Interpreting labels can be difficult, especially when it comes to understanding mineral needs. The above RDA for calcium is **expressed in milligrams of "elemental" calcium. The elemental calcium is the same as usable calcium.** For example, if a calcium supplement lists the contents as "calcium citrate = 950 mg." look carefully at the label to see how many milligrams of "calcium" or "elemental" calcium are in the product. If the label says, Calcium (elemental) = 200mg, that is the amount of calcium the supplement provides. This is true of all minerals. It is the "elemental" iron or "elemental" zinc that is usable.

[109] Cottage cheese has very little calcium. Low or non-fat cheeses are an excellent compromise for the cheese lover, and should be substituted for regular cheese whenever possible.

POTASSIUM

Potassium is an important nutrient found predominantly inside cells. This element along with sodium, is necessary for electrical impulses to travel along cell membranes. Electrical impulses in body cells are affected by too little or too much potassium. Low potassium causes muscle weakness and heart disturbances while a higher blood potassium could be toxic to the heart. Potassium helps lower blood pressure. A higher potassium, lower sodium diet is helpful in the control and prevention of hypertension. Although most Americans consume excessive sodium, the typical diet is low in potassium. Adults require about 3000[110] mg of dietary potassium daily. While half a cantaloupe contains 1000 mgs of potassium, and some fruit juices are excellent sources, many children, adolescents and adults consume drinks such as Kool Aid (containing only 1 mg of potassium), cola drinks (7 mg of potassium) coffee (40 mg of potassium), or beer (36 mg of potassium) instead. Simultaneously the hundred of milligrams of sodium contained in these drinks drives potassium out of balance. This combination of excess sodium and insufficient potassium contributes to the development of hypertension.

Hypertensive people who take diuretics lose potassium in their urine along with the sodium. Fatigue is the most common symptom of chronic potassium deficiency. The resulting muscle weakness and fatigue may be gradual and the extent of weakness not fully appreciated until the problem has been corrected.

In childhood, the major causes of potassium deficiency are related to diarrhea and hormonal imbalances. Because potassium regulates heartbeat, adolescents and young adults on a

---

110 There is no RDA for potassium or Estimated Safe and Adequate Daily Dietary Intake. The adult recommendation of 3000 milligrams of potassium per day is based on guidelines established by various health organizations and experts

prolonged weight losing diet consuming exclusively a low potassium "liquid protein diet" or those with anorexia nervosa can have a very low heart rate and become gravely ill. Maintaining consistent levels of potassium in the blood and cells is vital to body function.

Potassium is found in a large range of foods, especially oranges, bananas, potatoes (with skin), apricots, prunes, tomatoes, whole grains, legumes, meats, and fish.

MAGNESIUM

Magnesium is an important mineral in human nutrition and shares many of the attributes of calcium. Its distribution in the body is much the same as potassium. Magnesium, calcium and potassium control the body fluid and keep it from becoming too alkaline or acidic. Magnesium is an integral part of bone crystal, and it activates enzymes for hundreds of reactions including those that involve the expenditure of energy. It is a component of chlorophyll and is also found in animal protein. Good sources of magnesium can be found in whole grains, legumes, dark leafy greens, vegetables, baked potatoes, beans, bananas, apricots, tuna and salmon.

Because it is found in so many foods and is abundant in nature, magnesium deficiency is extremely rare in healthy people. Deficiencies are mostly seen in alcoholism, persons with diabetes, kidney diseases, and from certain medications. Average consumption from our food is around 300 mg a day.[111]

Young, weight conscious women appear more susceptible to magnesium deficiency. This may be explained by the common use of diuretics, known to cause deficiency. Liquid protein diets

---

[111] Researchers at the National Cardiovascular Center in Osaka, Japan found that daily magnesium supplements of 480 mg decreased blood pressure in Japanese adults with high blood pressure.

are also associated with magnesium deficiency. Along with this loss is a loss of potassium, and a type of potassium deficiency that is difficult to correct.

Grand mal seizures, muscular weakness, heart muscle damage, and heart irregularities are some of the more severe consequences of magnesium deficiency.

CHLORINE (CHLORIDE)

Chlorine is extremely important in electrolyte balance and is a necessary component of gastric juice. Salt is the main provider of chloride in the body. Chloride also aids in the conservation of potassium and while dietary deficiency states are rare, in childhood it can be caused by chronic vomiting and in adults by the overuse of diuretic drugs. Many years ago a soybean-based infant formula was removed from the market after it was discovered to contain excessively low amounts of chloride. Some infants consuming this product early in infancy when no other foods were offered, developed symptoms ranging from marked irritability to severe growth failure. There was no outside source of chloride from solid foods for these infants to correct this deficiency. Catastrophes such as this demonstrate how dangerous it is to rely on a single food to provide all our nutrients, and points to the danger of fad diets, such as total milk, fruit, and high protein, or "liquid protein diets."

In the late 1960's, Dr. Joseph M. Price published his hypothesis claiming chlorine to be the major cause of cardiovascular disease. He pointed to chlorination of water supply as the origin of heart attacks. To support his argument he compared the lack of chlorination of water in China, Japan and parts of Kenya to places where it was present. His figures pointed to a direct relationship between the amount of chlorine consumed and the rate of heart attacks. Advocates of this hypothesis have prepared graphs of "surveys" to support these contentions as reasonable.

The adage, "figures don't lie, but liars figure," comes to mind when data is presented regardless of the source. In spite of my skepticism I have been caught many times blindly accepting information on face value because a study was performed by a reputable investigator at a prestigious institution. **Careful measurements that are reproducible** come slowly and with difficulty but are extremely important if we are to avoid embracing every wild claim by both charlatan and scientist.

The chlorine theory has been studied and despite claims of conspiracy that chlorine is a "sacred cow" of the establishment, there is no valid statistical evidence to support these claims. Careful statistical studies have not shown a significant relationship between chlorine intake and heart attack rates.

Our drinking water must be guarded against contamination from industrial waste at all costs, but chlorination of our water supply is not only safe, it protects us from water borne disease capable of causing severe illness. There is a theoretical risk from drinking chlorinated water. Chlorine is known to react with organic material and other pollutants to form traces of chloroform. Chloroform is a carcinogen, and there has been a study linking the presence of chloroform in the water supply to a slightly higher incidence of certain cancers. According to a February, 1998 study published in the medical journal, Epidemiology, from the California Department of Health Services, a contaminant, trihalomethanes,[112] (THM) commonly found in

[112] Trihalomethanes, (THM) are a family of chemicals formed during the chlorination process used in most municipal water systems nationwide. Trihalomethanes form when chlorine reacts with organic matter or with components of sea water. The EPA has been considering a stricter standard for trihalomethanes because exposure to the contaminant has also been linked to an increased risk of cancer. The study was led by Waller and Shanna Swann, an epidemiologist with the state Department of Health Services. The EPA helped fund the study.

chlorinated drinking water may be linked to a higher risk of miscarriage among pregnant women who drink five or more glasses of tap water a day. The study found that pregnant women in their first trimester who drank at least five glasses of tap water a day were roughly twice as likely to have a miscarriage as women who drank less water or whose water had lower concentrations of the contaminant. Health officials said they were taking the results seriously, but stressed that the findings are not definite and need to be confirmed by further research. There is also an association between THMs with the higher occurrence of "Small For Gestational Age" (SGA) infant births. Some health officials recommended that pregnant women find alternatives to unfiltered tap water, such as bottled water.

Despite the undisputed benefits of chlorination in controlling waterborne infectious diseases, the epidemiologic evidence now available suggests that chlorination disinfection by-products (CBPs) may also play a causal role in human bladder cancer.

Monitoring and controlling levels of CBPs in our water supply is an important public health issue and must not be ignored.

I enjoy bottled water because of taste, but many people choose bottled water because of a fear of their municipal water supply. The water supply in the United States is probably one of the safest in the world, but to keep it so, constant vigilance and support are needed to safeguard our most precious resource. **If you use well water, be sure to have it tested for safety.**

Think of all of those "throw away" plastic bottles contaminating the oceans and waterways. Non-disposable glass containers filled with CBPs free water and kept in the refrigerator are healthier for the environment as well.

"IONIZED" AND ALKALINE WATER"

I will not go into this pseudoscientific absurdity ready made for the most gullible (often characterized as "open-minded").

For those interested in this matter, I refer you to the website: www.chem1.com/CQ/ionbunk.html. and www.quackwatch.org.

One more word about drinking water, that is, ice water with a meal. You may have been advised not to drink ice water with a meal. The explanation is that it damages your body's ability to properly digest food and drink. So instead, food goes by improperly digested and the body is unable to retrieve the nutrients and energy from it that it needs. By decreasing the activity of your digestive system, they claim cold beverages rob you of the nutrition of the food and your body has to use energy in order to warm up that liquid inside your body. These pseudo-nutritionists proclaim further, without a shred of evidence, that the immune system, which works to fight off colds and other illnesses, can also suffer from this poor digestion because it does not have the energy it needs to function correctly.

The lack of critical thinking skills and the naivety of those who, without looking for a scientific source for this hypothesis, blindly accepts such humbug . This reveals their gullibility and how poorly they understanding evidence based science.

IRON

Iron deficiency is one of the most widespread nutritional deficiency problems still seen in the United States. Although there is much written about other minerals and vitamins allegedly being in short supply in our diet, iron deficiency remains a real problem in infancy, adolescence, and especially in pregnancy.

When one thinks of iron deficiency, anemia is the problem that often comes to mind. But depletion of body stores of iron causes many problems long before anemia or low hemoglobin occurs, such as irritability and poor appetite in children. By the time anemia is present, other behavioral changes such as pica and craving for ice frequently occur. It has been suggested that ice craving can occasionally cause alcoholism since it is socially acceptable for adults to drink ice with alcoholic drinks. Allegedly the iron deficient compulsive ice eater gets habituated to the alcohol as well. Treatment with iron pills results in the disappearance of ice craving, poor appetite, and irritability usually within a week, and long before the iron deficiency itself is corrected. Chronic fatigue is believed to be a relatively late symptom in iron deficiency, but decreased work performance has been found in people with even mild iron deficiency.

Doctors test for anemia with a simple hemoglobin test. The results might appear normal, and a patient may have no obvious illness, but iron deficiency may still exist. This is especially so during periods of rapid growth as during infancy, adolescence and throughout the childbearing period in women. During these times when demand for iron for hemoglobin formation and muscle is increased, additional iron is needed in the diet. Especially at risk are premature infants and children 6 months to 3 years of age. Regular aspirin users are also at high risk for iron deficiency. For these reasons iron fortification has been promoted by public health minded nutritionists. Rather than relying on people to remember to take extra iron every day in pill form, iron has been added to flour and cereal. For those who prefer to get their iron from more natural sources, good ones are whole wheat, fish, poultry (the dark has more iron than white meat), figs, dates, beans, asparagus, black strap molasses, oatmeal, enriched bread, dark green vegetables, and extra lean meat. One cup of prune juice supplies 55% of an adult woman's RDA for iron. Cooking in iron pots and pans contributes a great deal of extra iron to the diet. The much fabled spinach,[113] Popeye's ready source, has many milligrams of iron, but in the form of poorly absorbable iron oxalate. Even the iron in egg yolk may not be as absorbable as once thought. Broccoli has significantly more available iron (and calcium). Phosphates, found in sodas, also form compounds with iron which are difficult for the body

[113] Spinach is good for you. It is exceptionally high in beta carotene and folic acid.

to absorb. Some foods decrease iron absorption. Bran and teas containing tannin are two. (Coffee which contains no tannins, depresses absorption, but to a lesser degree.) More than a quart of milk a day also contributes to iron deficiency.

In contrast, other foods increase iron absorption, particularly vitamin C rich foods. The vitamin C counteracts the effects of other iron inhibitors. The vitamin C changes the poorly absorbable ferric iron found in many foods to the more soluble ferrous form. Vitamin C, however, is not an important enhancer of iron pill absorption since it is already in the ferrous form. This is important to remember, especially for pregnant women, who are often advised to take high does of iron supplements. Taking a ferrous iron pill before breakfast insures excellent absorption. Small amounts of animal protein (non-dairy) such as beef, poultry, or fish added to a meal can increase iron absorption from food four fold.

Many people wish to take iron supplements[114] because of the fact that the bioavailability of iron in foods varies so greatly. In the ordinary diet 10-20 mg of iron are consumed each day, but less than 10% of this is absorbed. The requirements for iron found in the RDA take into account the low amount of iron actually absorbed from iron pills. I tell my patients that in recommended doses iron is safe, but to be careful not to consume too much iron as a supplement because in large amounts it can be toxic and cause abdominal discomfort. Ferrous sulfate is a good supplement to take if needed, as it is very well absorbed. Some chelated

[114] Hemochromatosis, one of the most common hereditary diseases in the United States, is a deadly genetic disease that causes the organs to store too much iron. It can cause liver damage, diabetes, sterility and is often a "silent"disease, causing no symptoms. Men over 50 are five times more likely than women to show symptoms of hemochromatosis. High iron levels have been found in young men in their 20's and 30's. It can be detected by laboratory tests called "ferritin" and "transferrin saturation"blood levels. Ask your doctor to test you for hemochromatosis. Adult men should avoid iron supplements unless they need iron and are certain they do not have hemochromatosis.

iron compounds which are sold because of its less irritating effect on the gut, are often passed out in the stool without being utilized.

Infant formulas should have 12-18 mg of iron per quart. Breast fed infants get iron from breast milk in adequate amounts because of its extremely high bioavailability. Fortified infant cereals should not be feared. They are especially nutritious and contain the type of additives that are nutritionally desirable. Premature infants especially, if not breastfed, should be on an iron fortified formula.

Heavy menstrual periods are a frequent contributor to iron deficiency, which is why women after puberty and during child-bearing years are frequently iron deficient. It is very popular now for many men and women to totally avoid red meat. Women who avoid red meat are especially vulnerable to iron deficiency without obvious symptoms and might benefit from a small daily iron supplement. It is extremely rare for an adult man to be anemic due to lack of iron. Anemia in adult men should always be thoroughly investigated for its cause. Taking iron tablets could hide and postpone early diagnosis or recognition of blood loss in the stools from colitis, polyps, kidney disease or intestinal cancer.

RECOMMENDED DAILY ALLOWANCES FOR IRON[115]

Infants	**0-6 months**	**10 mg**
6 months to 3 years	**15 mg**	
Children	**4-10 years**	**10 mg**
Males & Females	**11-18 years**	**18 mg**
Males	**19 & over**	**10 mg**
Females	**19-50 years**	**18 mg**
51 & over	**10 mg**	
Pregnancy	**36 mg**	
Lactation (breastfeeding mothers)		**18 mg**

115 Individual requirements vary greatly; increasing the dietary iron through fortification may be desirable, particularly during pregnancy.

The above RDA for Iron is expressed in milligrams of "elemental" iron. The elemental iron is the same as usable iron. For example, there are 220 mg of ferrous sulfate in one teaspoon of the elixir (liquid form) and this equals 50 mg of elemental iron. The usual tablet of ferrous sulfate is 325 mg, but it delivers 65 mg of elemental iron.

ZINC

In 1963, zinc was first recognized as an essential element for humans. A normal American diet easily supplies the RDA for zinc because most Americans eat animal protein and zinc is found in abundant amounts in all meats. Diets which exclude meat, fish and other zinc rich foods such as eggs, milk and whole grains, may produce symptoms of zinc deficiency. Deficiency is also a potential problem in alcoholics with liver disease, patients with chronic kidney disease, rheumatoid arthritis, inflammatory bowel disease, and malabsorption syndrome (nutrients poorly absorbed from the gut). The rash that is characteristic of zinc deficiency resembles eczema. It occurs on the face, hands, feet and ano-genital regions. Other signs of zinc deficiency are loss of appetite, loss of taste, and possibly slower wound healing. These symptoms can also appear in individuals following an unusual crash diet.

At the opposite end of the spectrum is zinc toxicity due to zinc overdose (As with zinc deficiency, this is extremely rare, except in cases in which a person has been taking large zinc supplements and has a diet which is already high in zinc). Sometimes zinc poisoning (toxicity) is due to the ingesting foods stored in galvanized containers. Water that flows through galvanized pipes does not pose a problem, however. Symptoms of zinc toxicity are stomach upset, nausea, vomiting, bleeding in the stomach, and anemia secondary to this blood loss. Long term zinc overdose[116] can also interfere with resistance to infection.

Zinc deficiency in humans was first reported in the early 1960's in very short individuals found to be on a diet low in meat and fish, but very high in bread made from grains high in phytates. Phytates are known to bind zinc and thus inhibit its uptake in the body. Upon treatment with supplemental zinc these patients showed a striking response in growth and development of their secondary sex characteristics. Immediate responses to zinc supplementation in **deficient** persons include personality changes, clearing of skin lesions as well as increased body growth, particularly in infants. Children with zinc deficiency are extremely irritable and difficult to manage. The first response to zinc supplementation in deficient young children is that they become more placid, usually within 24 hours after the first treatment.

Recently, intriguing studies have suggested that zinc lozenges, when started within 24 hours of symptoms, may be effective in reducing the symptoms and duration of the common cold by up to 42%. A study[117] showed that if zinc lozenges were started with 24 hours of onset of cold symptoms, and administered no less than two hours apart (up to eight lozenges per day) cold symptoms lasted only 4.3 versus the 9.2 days found in a matched placebo group. Researchers aren't sure how zinc affects the common cold but they do know that in a test tube, zinc stops many cold viruses from multiplying. To date more than 300 zinc-dependent enzymes have been identified, thus promoting multiple theories on how zinc might work in preventing the common cold. It may induce the production of

[116] Large doses of zinc can interrupt the function of iron, aggravate a marginal copper deficiency and potentially contribute to calcium deficiency. Since all nutrients have the ability to influence the absorption of others, supplementation with any single vitamin or mineral, when taken in large amounts, is often not a good idea.

[117] Ann Intern Med 1996; 125(2):81-8.

interferon or the effect may be due in part to correction of subclinical zinc deficiency in selected persons. There is no shortage of theories! Whatever the mechanism, these recent studies raise the intriguing possibility that zinc may be effective in reducing the duration and severity of the common cold. Unfortunately, zinc is not always well tolerated. Ninety percent of those taking zinc lozenges (23 mg of elemental zinc usually as zinc gluconate) reported mild to moderate side effects such as nausea and bad taste.

Carefully conducted studies are needed before this therapy can be recommended, especially to children. If zinc becomes a widely used remedy against the common cold, long term surveillance will be necessary to verify its safety.[118] Much of the commercial hype about zinc's ability to prevent or modify the common cold is overstated.

THE RECOMMENDED DIETARY ALLOWANCE FOR ZINC

	RDA
Infants 0-12 months	**5 mg**
Children 1-10 years old	**10 mg**
Males 11-51+	**15 mg**
Females 11-51+	**12 mg**
Pregnancy	**15 mg**
Lactation 1st 6 months	**19 mg**
2nd 6 months	**16 mg**

[118] Zinc toxicity has been seen in people who took just 10 times the RDA of 15 mg zinc for several weeks.

FLUORIDE

When communities began to add fluoride to of drinking water in the 1960's, rates in tooth decay fell by 50 to 60 percent. Fluoride strengthens tooth enamel, making it more resistant to acids formed in the mouth by sugar fermenting bacteria. For those children living outside of water districts that fluoridate their water, fluoride drops or pills are almost as effective as drinking fluoridated water. But even the most motivated parent knows it is difficult to remember to give a child that daily fluoride pill for ten or more years. Parents often are more motivated to give a daily multivitamin to their child, so fluoride is often prescribed combined with a multivitamin and these preparations work as well as if they were given separately. Fluoride given on an empty stomach is 100% absorbed, but when given with milk or a calcium rich meal, it is incompletely absorbed. Fluoridated tooth paste is very popular and is of value in reducing caries. Very little tooth paste is needed to brush teeth adequately, and since many young children swallow toothpaste, it is prudent to keep the amount of paste to a small bead. Too much fluoride can cause slight mottling of the tooth enamel. The risk of mottling can be reduced by carefully following the current recommended supplementation dosages by the American Academy of Pediatrics Committee on Nutrition. Fluoride also favors the deposition of calcium, thereby strengthening bones and may help prevent osteoporosis. This has not been substantiated in large studies. The safety and nutrition advantages that result from fluoridation of the water supply have been demonstrated, but there are those who feel our water supply should not be tampered with. Although the argument for "freedom of choice" may be valid, the scare tactics used by anti-fluoridationists are unsupported by reputable studies. The amount added–one part fluoride to one million parts of water–does not cause cancer, nor is fluoridation a foreign plot to weaken our children's bodies, as some claim.

Breast milk, cow milk, prepared infant foods, beverages, and sodas contain virtually no fluoride. Various food snacks have been graded for their cavity producing capacity. Snack raisins are the worst, followed by cookies, sticky candy bars, doughnuts, and pre-sweetened cereals; then nut butters, chips and soda pop. While on the subject of tooth decay, I would be remiss not to mention fruit juices. Fruit juice is pure sugar. That's right–natural sugar, but nonetheless sugar. I frequently observe parents giving three bottles of juice a day to their infants and toddlers to use as a pacifier. This means that

the child washes his or her teeth with sugar constantly, which leads to "apple juice teeth." It need not be apple juice, it can be any fruit juice or even cow or breast milk (they contain the milk sugar, lactose). In addition to tooth decay, the sugar in fruit juice often is responsible for a poor appetite and results in a very irritable child. Limit juice to once a day and if you must use the "bottle" as a pacifier, **fill it with pure water, and not dilute juice.**

Supplementation of the diet is no substitute for a wholesome diet. To achieve and maintain healthy teeth and gums throughout life, oral hygiene, optimal nutrition, and avoidance of sticky snacks are critical.

FLUORIDE SUPPLEMENTATION SCHEDULE

∑ **No supplementation for water containing over 0.6 ppm fluoride**

∑ **No supplementation for infants under six months of age.**

∑ **No supplementation for children under three years of age where fluoride level is over 0.3 ppm.**

Discuss with your dentist whether there is a need to supplement with fluoride or if periodic dental application is sufficient.

SELENIUM

Recent studies suggest that selenium might be involved in a variety of important biological processes, including those of the immune system. Animal studies have demonstrated that selenium offers some protection against environmental carcinogens. Selenium is one of a group of minerals including zinc, copper, iron, and manganese all of which help neutralize free radicals. That is, they help fight cell damage caused by oxygen derived compounds; and thus may protect against certain cancers. For these reasons, it has been recommended that malnourished people take selenium as a supplement up to a maximum of 50 micrograms a day. However, selenium can also be quite toxic and the range between safe and too much is very narrow.

In the general population, dietary selenium intake varies greatly, depending on the type of food consumed and the geographic location in which these foods are produced. Selenium is not distributed evenly in agricultural lands. As a result, many of our foods are grown in selenium deficient soils. Since selenium is not essential for the growth of grains, fertilizers usually do not contain selenium. In the USA and Canada it has been reported that the more selenium found in the soil and farm crops, the lower the human cancer rate in those areas.

Keshan disease is a potentially fatal heart muscle and muscle weakness disease found in young children deficient in selenium. It is seen in China where selenium is deficient in the soil. It is occasionally seen in premature infants kept on intravenous fluids for weeks when the nutrient fluid has no added selenium. Selenium supplementation programs in China have eradicated this widespread problem.

Fortunately, seafood, especially oysters, halibut, swordfish, salmon, and tuna, is rich in selenium and is an excellent low fat source of protein as well. Other foods rich in selenium include yeast, asparagus, garlic, whole grains, and cashews. Although kelp is rich in selenium, many other toxic metals such as arsenic and mercury may also be present.

COPPER

Copper is an essential nutrient which the body stores in the liver. It is crucial to respiration, hemoglobin synthesis, bone and connective tissue growth, and normal function of the central nervous system. There are several extremely rare causes of copper deficiency at birth that have to do with genetic inborn errors of metabolism (Wilson's disease, Menke's disease). Copper deficiency due to inadequate intake of this mineral is primarily seen in patients fed for long periods on intravenous fluid deficient in this mineral. An early feature of nutritional copper deficiency is anemia unresponsive to iron therapy. Large quantities of supplemental zinc can also impair copper absorption. On a practical level, copper deficiency should not be a concern to parents.

Good dietary sources of copper are shellfish, (especially oysters),[119]beans, nuts, whole grains and potatoes.

IODINE

Iodine is needed for normal cell metabolism and for the thyroid gland to make thyroid hormones. Insufficient intake of this trace element can lead to a goiter due to enlargement of the thyroid gland. Goiters were once common in parts of the world, called "goiter belts," where the soil was deficient in iodine. In the United States, the goiter belt included the Great Lakes region and the Plain states. In the 1930's about 40% of the people in Michigan had a goiter due mainly to iodine deficiency. As a public

[119] Raw or uncooked shellfish is dangerous at any age, but especially in the very young and old. It is safer and wiser to consume only cooked, steamed, barbecued, or baked shellfish and crustaceans.

health measure, iodized salt was introduced, and although we still see goiters in America, they are rarely due to iodine deficiency.

Cretinism, a form of mental retardation, is found in infants born with little or no thyroid hormone and was once commonly caused by iodine deficiency. The mental retardation of cretinism can be prevented by giving these infants thyroid hormone immediately after birth. Most newborns in the United States are screened by a blood test to help obtain an early diagnosis of this preventable disaster.

In a recent study that appeared in the medical Journal Lancet, mild to moderate iodine deficiency in pregnancy is linked to lower IQ in offspring. Worse effects were seen among women with severe deficiency than those with mild to moderate deficiency. The authors advise that pregnant and breastfeeding women take prenatal vitamins containing iodine.

The best sources of iodine are iodized salt, seafood, and dairy products and crops grown from iodine rich areas. It is extremely unlikely that iodine deficiency would occur in children or adults on a low salt diet, since only minuscule amounts are needed -micrograms- and therefore supplementation is rarely needed. Most multivitamin-mineral supplements contain 150 mcg.

RECOMMENDED DAILY ALLOWANCE FOR IODINE

	(RDA in mcg)
Infants	**40-50**
1-3 years	**70**
4-6 years	**90**
7-10 years	**120**
11 and older	**150**
Pregnancy	**175**
Lactation	**200**

THE FOOD GUIDE PYRAMID NOW BECOMES A "PLATE"

▲ ▲ ▲

A GUIDE TO DAILY FOOD CHOICES

The Food Pyramid was a visual model of what constituted a healthy diet. It was divided into many sections, each representing a food group with the largest section at its base. Foods in that section made up the largest part of your adult diet. As one got to the top of the pyramid the sections become smaller, suggesting smaller portions of the daily diet should be consumed from this group. The smallest section at the top of the pyramid represented Fats, Oils and Sweets, and the advice was to use these foods sparingly, that is, 1-2 tablespoons of added fat a day and 2-6 tablespoons of added sugar a day! This was of limited value for children. The size of food servings were more appropriate for adults and there was little to warn the parent against hidden fats, sugars or salt. After looking at the recommended portion size for vegetables, parents might correctly wonder, "What child would eat all of that?" Obviously, serving sizes had to be scaled down for children, especially those under ten.

Each section contained pictures of foods which afforded quick identification of the "healthy" foods. A clever promoter could place a picture or icon of his food, suggesting its wholesomeness. For example, the bottom section is for grains, primarily unprocessed, - Bread, Cereals, Rice, and Pasta - instead, products such as pizza with cheese, olives, and pepperoni toppings or a box of macaroni & cheese might be displayed.

The Milk, Yogurt, and Cheese section near the top of the pyramid did not stress non-or low fat dairy. If you followed the portion size of recommended servings within this group plus the adjacent Meat, Poultry, Fish, Dry Beans, Eggs & Nuts group, you and your children most likely would be eating excessive amounts of protein, sugar and fat.

That two thirds of the FOOD PYRAMID was devoted to the complex carbohydrate. This was supposed to serve as visual reminder that whole grains, fresh vegetables and fruit should be the most prominent part of each meal, while only one third or less of your plate should be covered with the meat, poultry, fish, cheese or eggs. This message redeemed the other flaws, but clearly, this Pyramid needed work.

Now the USDA, the agency in charge of nutrition, has switched to a new symbol: a colorful plate called, "My Plate" with the same message.

The Plate features four sections-vegetables, fruits, grains, and protein plus a side order of dairy. The big message is that fruits and vegetables take up half the plate, with the vegetable portion being a little bigger than the fruit section. The grain section is bigger than the protein section because it is recommended you eat more vegetables than fruit and more grains than animal protein foods. The divided plate also aims to discourage super-big portions, which can cause overweight.

Keep up to date on how the USDA's MyPlate can help you and your family's food choices by checking new tools at: www.ChooseMyPlate.gov

Serving Size

COMPLEX CARBOHYDRATES THE FOUNDATION OF THE PLATE

Grains, rice, potatoes, pasta, bread, tortillas, couscous, quinoa, polenta :

A child's serving size is 1/3 the adult portion

1 cup cooked spaghetti approximates the size of an adult fist

1 cup mashed potato approximates the size of an apple

More examples of foods found in the category are:

High fiber muffins, grits, cornbread, corn, wheat, quinoa, rye or oat cereals should be easy to find. Select dry cereals and crackers with three or more grams of fiber per serving. More difficult to find might be high fiber pasta or bagels. Combine any low fiber grain-foods with fiber rich spreads such as hummus instead of high fat cream cheese. Use a low fat high fiber vegetable sauce as a topping for macaroni or spaghetti. Use the highest fiber rice available to you, such as brown rice and try to avoid the highly processed "instant rice." Eat the skin of baked or boiled potatoes to increase the fiber and mineral content.

Children love crackers. It's true that they are a grain, but most have had much of the nutrition removed and replaced with too much sodium and fat. Select crackers higher in fiber

as recommended in THE MARIN COUNTY DIET: Feed Your Child RIGHT From Birth.

Other grains to avoid are dehydrated Ramen soups. The fiber has been removed from the noodles and to make things worse, the noodles are fried. These products also contain excess sodium and may have MSG. Most boxed macaroni and cheese should not be listed as an acceptable grain for similar reasons.

Many foods, such as milk, pizza, soups, sandwiches are combinations of complex carbohydrates, fats, proteins and simple sugars. That's why we need the

Nutritional Facts along with MY PLATE.

MORE COMPLEX CARBOHYDRATES FRUITS AND VEGETABLES

A child's serving size is one tablespoon per year of age or the adult serving, whichever works best for a particular food. A two year old serving size would be _ banana or pear, while using the tablespoon method, it would be two tablespoons of fruit or vegetable:

Vegetables: Carrots, squash, yams, peas, broccoli, Brussels sprouts, string-beans, spinach, Swiss chard, lettuce, celery, cucumbers, tomatoes, kale, and radishes.

Did I hear you say, "My children won't look at vegetables?" Then try soups.

Soups are an excellent delivery system for vegetables and most children love soups.

Fruit: Apple, banana, watermelon, kiwi, fig, orange, peach, pear, tangerine, grapefruit, plums, mango, cantaloupe, strawberries, blueberries and cherries. Fruit juice should be limited

to once a day at most. Better yet, once a week. Instead, eat the entire fruit, since it contains all that nutritional fiber and nutrients that are discarded during the juicing process.

PROTEIN FOODS
MEAT, FISH, POULTRY, EGGS, BEANS, TOFU, LENTIL AND DAIRY

This section contains low fat protein-rich food sources. Over the past sixty years, this group of foods has been over-consumed.

MILK[120] AND DAIRY

For a younger child, 2 cups of milk per day, is adequate. A child who fills up on milk has little room left over for other important foods such as fruits and vegetables.

ESTIMATING SIZE OF FOOD PORTIONS

One ounce of low-fat shredded mozzarella cheese approximates the size of a Ping-Pong ball.

One ounce of cubed low-fat Jack cheese approximates the size of 4 dice.

[120] One cup of milk is equal to one cup of yogurt or 1 1/2 oz. of low fat natural cheese.

MEATS, FISH, POULTRY, EGGS, BEANS, TOFU, LENTILS

A child's serving size is about an ounce. Keep in mind that the recommended adolescent or adult serving of meat is 2-3 ounces at a meal. A child under three years who takes 2 cups of milk plus one ounce of meat, beans, lentils, peas, fish or poultry, fulfills the RDA for protein. For children over 3 years, add one more ounce of a protein rich food.

3 oz. of beef or turkey breast approximates the size of a deck of cards.

Examples of protein found on MY PLATE are:
Fish (not fried), shrimp, eggs (not fried), low fat cheese, lean beef, turkey, lean pork, chicken (no skin and not fried), tofu, lentils, beans (not cooked with lard!), 1% or non-fat milk.

Remember that milk is a high protein food in addition to being an excellent calcium source. But dairy is very low in iron. If your family avoids red meat, (an excellent source of iron), because of philosophical or other reasons, be sure to eat iron fortified grains and cereals. Consider taking a daily iron supplement after consulting with your personal physician.

Do not overwhelm your child with a plate too full of food.

A small portion of MYPLATE contains "fun foods" or "holiday foods" and may be consumed on special occasions. They are not truly "foods" but are treats which add joy to the life of a child (or adult) as long as these foods are kept special. Historically, these foods were served on holidays, and when used in such a way, pose no long term nutritional problem. <u>But when packed away daily in the school lunch bag they become a health hazard.</u>

Examples found in this category are:

Ice cream, potato chips, French fries, fruit roll-ups, M & M's, Snicker Bars, "Sports Energy" bar, Fruit punches, pickles, hot dogs, sausage, liverwurst, lunch meats, chicken nuggets, smoked fish, butter, margarine, Caesar, Roquefort, mayonnaise, or other high fat dressings.

The extremely popular Combo Meal at McDonalds-a Big Mac, Medium Fries, and a soda provides 1,130 calories (for under $6:00) and 1380mg sodium, plus 19 teaspoons sugar. Do you really want this for your child, even at such a low price?

PART III

▲ ▲ ▲

THE MARIN COUNTY DIET

FEED YOUR CHILD RIGHT FROM BIRTH

RESOURCES FOR PARENTS

RECIPES

▲ ▲ ▲

STOCKING THE WHOLESOME KITCHEN
KITCHEN TOOLS FOR LOW-FAT COOKING

1. Set of non-stick cookware. This lets you sauté without butter, margarine, or oil. Also keep a can of non-stick spray on hand for baking pans or cookie sheets, if called for. Depending on how creative you want to get, non-stick muffin or cupcake pans, and a non-stick wok can also come in handy.

2. Air popcorn popper

3. Roasting rack so meat or poultry doesn't have to sit in its own fat while it cooks. Fat collects at the bottom of the pan and can be drained off after cooking.

4. Blender[121] or food processor for making purees, smoothies, sorbets, soups, shakes, and other drinks; as well as grating carrots, shredding cabbage, chopping celery, parsley, or cilantro. I like the Vita-Mixer-type juicers that don't remove the pulp.

[121] Vita-Mixer sold in many Costco stores

5. Electric mixer
6. Steamer basket
7. Plastic spatulas
8. Thick plastic cutting board (better than wood because it retards bacterial growth)
9. Zipper type bags
10. Microwave oven. They're safe and very helpful in preparing low-fat meals at a moment's notice. Microwave cooking destroys fewer vitamins than other methods of cooking

KITCHEN CONDIMENTS AND STAPLES FOR THE CUPBOARD AND REFRIGERATOR

1. Herbs, especially fresh herbs, enhance the flavor of foods and allow you to reduce or eliminate salt.
2. No-sodium-added condiments (as in ketchup), herbal salt substitutes, sodium-free seasonings, lemon juice, no salt added tomato juice (Even if you add a little salt to "improve" the flavor, it will still be less than the regular tomato juice.), garlic cloves, onions, cocoa instead of chocolate, non or low-fat sour cream,[122] non or low fat mayo, non or low fat plain yogurt, vinegar, virgin olive oil, canola oil, a plastic bottle of I Can't Believe It's Not Butter Spray (great flavoring and only 2 grams of fat in 18 spritzes), fat free chicken broth (All Natural-KITCHEN

[122] Some brands of non-fat sour cream have a poor taste, but many others are excellent. Check the different brands at your local market and don't stop looking if your first selection was not to your liking.

BASICS unsalted Chicken Cooking Stock or Progresso's 100% Unsalted CHICKEN BROTH.

3. Fat free or low saturated fat muffin and pancake mixes. Saturated fat free reduced sugar fudge brownie or angel food cake mix. (beware of the sugar added to take the place of the fat!) Whole grain breads.

4. Low fat or non-fat salad dressings. Low fat or non-fat mayonnaise[123]. Fresh salsa.

5. Pre-cut, pre-chopped, bagged greens and pre-cut veggies, such as broccoli, cauliflower, and carrots, make salad preparation a breeze; Box of cherry tomatoes; Low sodium dip mixes such as Knorr (make with nonfat sour cream).

6. Boil-in-the bag rice, white or brown, for always perfect rice without having to use the highly processed and totally defibered instant rice. A bag of small new or red potatoes, potatoes for baking or microwaving. A can of fat-free refried beans for a high fiber burrito or as a dip.

7. Low saturated fat, low sodium, low sugar breakfast cereals that are high in fiber and vitamins. A few examples are: Uncle Sam original, Cheerios, Kellogg's Bran Flakes, Barbara's Shredded Wheat, Kashi Go Lean, and Organic Cooked Brown Rice in a cup.

8. One percent or non-fat milk (for children over 2 years), but <u>not the 2% "low fat" milk which is not really low in fat.</u>

9. Seasonal, <u>ripe</u> fresh fruit. Do not buy fruit that was prematurely picked and is hard as a rock. It you discover when you get home that the fruit tastes like cardboard, return it to your grocer. (I ripen fresh fruit that is still hard by keeping it in the trunk of my card for 3-4 days)

[123] Best Foods Low Fat Mayo has an excellent flavor.

10. Apple sauce with no sugar added and no HFCS.
11. Whole Wheat Bagels, breadsticks, unsalted pretzels, matzo, whole wheat pita (pocket) bread, corn tortillas, non-fat whole wheat tortillas, popcorn for an air popcorn popper, fat free fig bars, dried fruit, assorted nuts, rice cakes, low sodium water-packed tuna, low fat or fat free string cheese, canned reduced salt black beans, and don't forget the Beano.
12. Dried spaghetti, linguini, macaroni, angel hair pasta. Non or low-fat, reduced sodium marinara sauce.
13. Frozen skinless chicken breasts, Boca Burgers, Vegie-Burgers, extra-lean hamburger meat.
14. All-purpose flour.
15. Fresh easy to peel oranges or tangerines.

FOOD SHOULD NEVER BE LEFT AT ROOM TEMPERATURE FOR MORE THAN TWO HOURS. LEFTOVERS SHOULD BE PLACED IN SHALLOW CONTAINERS AND PUT DIRECTLY IN THE REFRIGERATOR OR FREEZER.

PREVENTION OF NUTRITIONAL LOSSES FROM FOODS

Storage, processing, and cooking of fresh vegetables can cause nutritional losses. As a generalization, minerals, carbohydrates, fats, protein, vitamin K, and niacin are stable (greater than 85% retention) during processing and storage of foods. The nutrients most affected by cooking at home are the B-complex vitamins and vitamin C because these vitamins dissolve in water and are usually drained away in the cooking water. Prolonged cooking in too much water as well as cutting vegetables into small pieces before cooking (processing) tend to increase vitamin loss. A basic rule for maintaining the nutrient is to cook vegetables in water which weighs no more than 1/3 as much as the food. For example, if you were to cook a pound of vegetables you would need only 1/3 of a pound of cooking water. One pound of water is equivalent to one pint, so 1/3 of a pound of water would amount to less than a cup. If cooking water does not cover the vegetable, steam from the boiling water will still cook it completely.

It is important to limit the cooking water only if it is to be discarded. If it is saved to be eaten in soup, it makes no difference--the vitamins remain.

To further reduce all vitamin losses, cook your food no longer than is necessary to suit your taste. Food should be cooked as soon before serving as possible since the nutritional value of food is highest at that time.

Steaming brings less water into contact with vegetables than boiling. But steam still wets the vegetables and the water drips back into the pan. Steaming and boiling in a small quantity of water are nearly equal in removing vitamins.

Microwaving is a rapid method of cooking and causes minimal vitamin loss.

Storage of cooked vegetables for a day or longer in the refrigerator and then reheated results in losses of vitamin C between 25 to 50%. Vitamins in foods are also destroyed when stored in the freezer. The colder the refrigerator or freezer, the smaller the loss will be. Concentrated frozen orange juice refrigerated one year loses only 5% of the vitamin C. As a rule, however, there can be a significant loss of nutritional value when a food is stored longer than a few months in the freezer. Freezing slows destruction of nutrients but does not completely stop the destruction.

Vitamin A is reasonably stable in almost all food products and processes, but a notable exception is dehydrated foods exposed to air. Extended cooking of green, yellow or red vegetables can lower the vitamin A by 15-35%, but cooking high fiber foods such as carrot probably increases the absorption of vitamin A.

Folic acid losses average only 10% during baking while prolonged cooking of meat destroys this B vitamin.

Vitamin D is sensitive to light and that is why milk should be stored in opaque containers such as cartons rather than clear glass bottles.

Tips to boost vitamins and minerals in your diet:

1. Purchase only the freshest vegetables and fruits because vitamins are lost when produce is wilted, bruised, or old.

2. Darker colored vegetables are generally richer in nutrients. Dark green salad leaves for example, provide more vitamin A and iron than lighter ones. Orange carrots have more vitamin A than paler, yellow carrots. **Yellow corn is more nutritious than white corn.**

3. Pay attention to "sell before" expirations dates on milk and cottage cheese containers. Select the "youngest" product to assure freshest flavor and best maintenance of B vitamins.

4. Avoid overcooking meat and fish. Medium or medium rare rather than well done meat or seafood contains more B-1 (thiamine). **An exception is hamburger meat. All ground meat should be cooked well done, to kill any contaminating bacteria.**

5. Refrigerate leftover vegetables as soon as possible and use them within a day or two.

6. Potatoes, onions, carrots, sweet potatoes keep best in a cool place (about 50 degrees F).

7. Ripen tomatoes at room temperature and then refrigerate when ripe. Use as soon as they are ripe because tomatoes lose vitamin C with aging.

8. Fresh vegetables should be used soon after purchase. Vitamins and flavor are lost when vegetables are kept too long in the refrigerator.

RECIPES

Complex Carbohydrate Recipes
Grains, Rice, Potatoes, Pasta, Bread, Tortillas, Couscous, and Poleta.

BASIC MASHED POTATOES

Serves 6

6 medium russet potatoes, washed
3/4 cup nonfat milk, warmed
Ground black pepper
Optional: salt, Butter Buds, salt substitute, nonfat yogurt, buttermilk, chives, scallions, nonfat chicken broth

Peel potatoes and cut into quarters. Put in a large saucepan and add enough water to cover them by about one inch. Bring water to a boil, reduce heat and simmer for about 20 minutes, or until potatoes are tender but not mushy. Drain well.

Mash potatoes with a potato masher or a mixer, and add warm nonfat milk (if using a mixer, don't over-mix or potatoes will be heavy). Gently stir in pepper to taste.

If desired, add a small amount of salt, Butter Buds, or a salt substitute when adding the pepper. For additional flavor, gently stir in any of the following: nonfat yogurt, buttermilk, chives, scallions, nonfat chicken broth.

BAKED POTATO

Russet potatoes are best for baking. Do not wrap them in foil, because the covering traps moisture, which will steam rather than bake the potatoes. Pierce the skin with a fork or knife in a few places before baking. This will permit the steam to escape, thus producing dry, fluffy potatoes. Thick-skinned potatoes may actually burst if baked without piercing. Baking nails can speed the baking process. Insert one lengthwise into each potato. Bake for 45-60 minutes in a 400 degree F oven. Test for doneness by squeezing the potato. It should give slightly. It's best to eat potatoes with their skins, which are rich in fiber,[124] iron, calcium, potassium, zinc, and B vitamins.

MICROWAVING POTATOES

Pierce the potatoes several times with a fork. Set them on a dish or double thickness of paper towel, placing a single potato in the center of the oven, and two or more in a circle or spoke pattern. Cooking times vary depending of the power of your microwave. Here are some stating suggestions. For one 8-oz potato allow 5 minutes: for two potatoes of the same size, 7 minutes; for 4 potatoes, 13 minutes. After removing them from the microwave, let them stand for 5 minutes before eating.

[124] Insoluable fiber, the kind in whole grains and beans, is thought to help prevent colon cancer and to reduce the risk of heart attacks in adults. This has not been confirmed by large controlled studies. Most nutritionists recommend an adult diet that includes 20-35 grams of fiber a day. That is the equivalent of two large bowls of wheat bran cereal. The average adult American consumes less than half that much. Sneaking fiber into the diet isn't difficult. For example, half a cup of blackberries contains about 2 grams of fiber while half a cup of blueberries contains 1 gram of fiber. Add berries to your cereal for the extra treat. For the child over four, air popped popcorn is another delicious source of nutritional fiber.

NEW POTATOES WITH DILL SAUCE

Serves 6

6 medium new potatoes, preferably red
Dill Sauce
4 ounces low fat or nonfat small curd cottage cheese
1/4 cup nonfat milk, warmed
1/2 teaspoon dry mustard
1/2 teaspoon prepared horseradish (not creamed)
1/2 teaspoon dried dill weed
Optional: 1/4 cup chives, 1/3 cup chopped scallions

Put potatoes in a large saucepan and add enough water to cover them by about one inch. Bring water to a boil, reduce heat and simmer for about 20 minutes or until potatoes are tender but not mushy. Drain well, allow to cool, and then slice into 1/4-inch rounds. Place in serving bowl and cover with dill sauce. Serve hot.

Make dill sauce while potatoes are boiling: blend cottage cheese and milk in a blender or food processor for about 30 seconds, until smooth and creamy. Transfer sauce to a small bowl and stir in dry mustard until dissolved. Add horseradish and dill weed and stir to combine. Chives or chopped scallions may be substituted for dill weed.

BAKED POTATO LATKE-TOTS

Recipe contributed by Mrs. Maddy Wilner

Makes about 36 Latke-Tots

3 large russet potatoes, peeled and grated
1 medium onion, peeled and grated
1/2 lemon, juiced
1 egg, beaten
2 tablespoons flour
1 teaspoon salt
1/2 teaspoon baking powder
1/2 teaspoon pepper
1 1/2 tablespoons canola oil
Vegetable oil cooking spray
Special equipment: non-stick mini muffin tin
Optional: powdered sugar, applesauce, nonfat sour cream

Preheat oven to 435°F.

Grate potatoes and onion in a food processor or with a hand grater. Transfer to a sieve and drain well. Add the grated potatoes and onions to a bowl and stir in the juice of the half lemon and the egg until well mixed.

Combine flour, salt, baking powder, and pepper and stir into the potato mixture. Add the canola oil, stirring to mix well.

Spray mini muffin tin generously with cooking spray and spoon potato mixture into each cavity, pressing gently to fill cavity. Bake in preheated oven for 20 to 25 minutes, until browned and crisp. Remove from oven and invert non-stick muffin tin onto a serving dish.

Serve hot with powdered sugar, apple sauce, or nonfat sour cream.

POTATO LATKES (PANCAKES)

Serves 6

3 medium russet potatoes, about 8 ounces each
1 medium onion, peeled
2 egg whites
1/2 lemon, juiced
1 to 2 tablespoons flour
2 teaspoons sugar
3/4 teaspoon baking powder
1/2 teaspoon salt
3 tablespoons canola oil, more if needed
Optional: applesauce, powdered sugar

Cut potatoes and onion into small pieces and add, with egg whites, to food processor or blender.[125] Pulse for about 25 to 30 seconds or until all chunks of potato are grated, but do not over-blend or your pancakes will not be the right texture. Transfer grated mixture into a large sieve and drain excess water. Put drained mixture in a large bowl and immediately stir in the lemon juice to prevent potatoes from oxidizing to a brown color. Add flour, sugar, baking powder and salt and mix thoroughly.

Heat a 10- or 12-inch non-stick skillet over medium heat and add enough oil (about 1 tablespoon) to coat the bottom of the pan. When oil is hot and forms a large bead add a heaping tablespoon of batter for each pancake and fry, covered, for 1 ½ minutes, tilting the pan to distribute the oil. Turn pancakes with a spatula and cook, covered, for another 2 to 4 minutes without adding more oil. When both sides of pancakes are golden brown

[125] Purists claim that a better latke is produced if the onion and potato are grated.

remove latkes to brown paper (such as a grocery bag) and allow the paper to absorb some of the oil.

Add a bit more oil to the pan (enough to coat the bottom) and follow the above instructions until the latke batter is gone. Serve immediately with applesauce, or with powdered sugar dusted over the top of each latke.

BASIC PREPARATION FOR VARIOUS KINDS OF RICE

All the recipes below call for 1 cup of dry rice with 2 cups of water. This makes about 3 cups of rice.

CONVERTED RICE: Although the directions on the box calls for 2-1/2 cups of water, use 2 cups. Bring the water to a boil in a pan and add the rice. Stir briefly. Cover and reduce heat to low. Do not disturb or remove cover. This means no peeking! Cook for 30 minutes. Remove cover and admire your perfect rice.

LONG GRAIN BROWN RICE: Bring the water to a boil and add rice. Mix briefly and cover. Reduce heat to low and simmer for 45 minutes. Don't remove cover until time's up!

WILD RICE: Same as above. When you uncover, if there's any unabsorbed water, drain it or let the rice stand uncovered for a few minutes.

Cooked rice will keep for about a week in the refrigerator. It reheats well if you add a few teaspoons of water. It is easy to vary the flavor of any rice by cooking it in a low or no-salt broth at the start and by adding spices or herbs such as parsley, cilantro, or dill to the freshly cooked grains. Substitute brown rice for pasta or use it as a base for shrimp, lean goulash, or stew. Pilaf is one of the most familiar rice dishes.

MEAT, RICE & KETCHUP

This dish was one of my children's' favorites for breakfast, lunch, dinner, or snack. It's nutritious and loved by children of all ages. Even my grandson, Cody, eats it.

Serves 4

1/2 pound extra lean ground beef
1 1/2 cups cooked white rice
1/2 cup ketchup
Green peas
Optional: 1/2 onion (chopped), 2 garlic cloves (minced), 1 1/2 teaspoons olive oil, red pepper flakes, ground black pepper

Heat a non-stick skillet over medium heat. Cook the ground beef until browned then tilt the pan and pour off any juices or fat. Stir in the rice and ketchup. Add a handful of green peas (thawed if frozen) and gently stir into beef.

For more sophisticated palates, sauté half a chopped onion and 2 garlic cloves in olive oil. Cook until soft and continue recipe as above. For spicier flavor add a pinch of red pepper flakes and some black pepper.

For those parents who want to prepare a quick rice dish, be sure to read the Nutrition Facts label before buying a box of a "ready to prepare" mix. Many are loaded with sodium. For example, the popular Rice-A-Roni Chicken & Vegetables has 1,470 mg of sodium in one small serving. The Center for Science in the Public Interest, Nutrition Action calls Rice-A-Roni "Rice-A-Salt," and recommends Marrakesh Express CousCous or Terrazza Pasta & Beans as healthier alternatives, because they cut out about 90% of the sodium.

POLENTA

Polenta is a corn mush made from corn flour. It's a staple among the poorer farmers in Europe and a fancy side dish among the upper classes in America. It's delicious for breakfast, lunch, dinner, or snacks.

Serves 2 to 3

1/2 cup polenta (or cornmeal)
2 cups water, divided
1/3 cup shredded reduced-fat or nonfat mozzarella or jack cheese
Optional: 1 teaspoon sugar

In a pot: Soak cornmeal for 15 minutes in ½ cup of water. Pour mixture into a pot of 1 1/2 cups boiling water. Reduce heat to low and simmer for 20 minutes. Stir constantly to avoid sticking or scorching. Add shredded cheese and stir into polenta until melted and well combined. Stir in the sugar if desired.

In a double boiler: The potential problem of sticking or scorching is avoided with a double boiler. Pour cornmeal slowly (to avoid lumping) into 2 cups of water in the top of a double boiler. Mix well and cook for about 35 minutes, stirring occasionally. Add shredded cheese and stir into polenta until melted and well combined. Stir in sugar if desired.

Variations: Polenta is often served with a sprinkling of Parmesan cheese, a spaghetti-meat sauce, Veracruzana Sauce (see recipe following), or with a chicken and tomato sauce dish.

VERACRUZANA SAUCE

Makes about 3 ½ cups

2 onions, thinly sliced and separated into rings
1 green bell pepper, quartered, seeded and cut crosswise into thin strips
2 garlic cloves, minced
1 can (16-ounces) low sodium tomatoes, or 2 cups chopped fresh tomatoes
1 can (4-ounces) pimientos
1 orange, juiced
1 dried red chili pepper, crushed
1 bay leaf
2 tablespoons fresh cilantro, or 1 teaspoon dried cilantro
1 tablespoon capers, drained
1/2 teaspoon dried oregano, crumbled
1/2 teaspoon ground cumin

Heat a non-stick skillet over medium heat and sauté onions until soft but not browned. Add green pepper and garlic and stir for 1 to 2 minutes. Break up tomatoes with a fork and add to skillet, along with remaining ingredients.

Bring to a boil, reduce heat and simmer, covered, for about 1 hour. May be cooled, then frozen in zip-style bags and stored for later use. This sauce is fantastic over chicken, rice, broiled red snapper or other white fish.

SPECIAL CREAM OF WHEAT®[126]

Serves 2 to 3

1 3/4 to 2 cups nonfat milk
1/3 cup Quick Cream of Wheat or Wheatena®[127]
2 egg whites
1 egg yolk (optional)
1 tablespoon brown sugar
1/2 teaspoon vanilla extract
Optional: raisins

Bring milk to a rapid boil over medium-high heat and slowly add Cream of Wheat or Wheatena,** stirring constantly. Return milk to a boil, reduce heat and cook for 2 1/2 minutes, or until thickened, stirring frequently.

Whisk the egg whites (and yolk, if desired) in a small bowl with the brown sugar and vanilla. Stir egg mixture into the Wheatena or Cream of Wheat and simmer for one more minute, stirring constantly. Add raisins if desired.

[126] Wheatena is a whole grain cereal while Cream of Wheat (farina) is mostly refined grain. There are more nutrients in whole grain cereals. Besides providing fiber as an aid in preventing constipation, whole grains are more likely to provide the vitamins, minerals, phytoestrogens, lignans, antioxidants and other unknown factors that are lost when grains are refined.

[127] You can also use an inexpensive metal steamer that fits inside a pan and suspends the vegetables over the water.

BUCKWHEAT PANCAKES

Makes 6 to 8 pancakes

1/2 cup rolled oats
1/4 cup buckwheat flour
1/4 teaspoon baking soda
1/4 teaspoon baking powder
1/2 cup nonfat yogurt
1/2 cup buttermilk
1 tablespoon apple juice concentrate
1 teaspoon vanilla extract
2 egg whites, stiffly beaten
Nonfat milk, if needed for thinning batter

Crushed fruit or berries

In a large bowl, combine oats, buckwheat flour, baking soda and baking powder and mix well. Add yogurt, buttermilk, apple juice concentrate and vanilla and combine thoroughly. Gently fold the beaten egg whites into the batter, thinning with a bit of milk if necessary.

Heat a non-stick griddle or skillet over medium-high heat and add about 1/4 cup batter for each pancake (pancakes will be about six-inches in diameter). Pour batter quickly onto griddle and lower heat slightly. Cook about 1 1/2 minutes per side, turning the pancakes when small air bubbles break on the top, then cooking until bottoms of pancakes are lightly browned.

Serve with crushed fresh fruit or berries on top. Maple syrup is also popular as a pancake topping, but fresh fruit and berries add more fiber and vitamins.

The Log Cabin Brand Maple Syrup had a seductive advertising gimmick when I was a child. The container was the shape of a long cabin. I'd beg my mother to buy that brand so I could play with the empty container. When she wasn't looking I'd pour some of the syrup in the sink to empty it more quickly. The syrup was too sweet and I really didn't like it very much. Remember that the body treats this as any other pure sugar.

QUICK OATMEAL

Serves 3 to 4

1 1/2 cups water
2/3 cup oatmeal (1-minute variety)
1/2 apple, chopped
1/4 cup raisins
1/2 teaspoon cinnamon
Optional: nonfat milk, banana slices

In a small saucepan bring water to a boil over medium-high heat and stir in oatmeal. Immediately reduce heat to medium-low and stir exactly 1 minute. Cover with tightly fitting lid, remove from heat, and allow to stand for 3 to 4 minutes. Add remaining ingredients and stir gently. May serve with nonfat milk or banana slices if desired.

KASHA VARNISHKAS

No guarantees for this recipe since it has not been kid-tested outside of Russia. If you are adventuresome and enjoy different tastes this might be a bright new addition to your repertoire.

This is traditionally served as a side dish with a meat course.

Serves 4 to 6

1 egg
1 cup kasha (buckwheat groats)
4 teaspoons canola or extra-virgin olive oil, divided
1 large onion, chopped
1 1/2 cups low sodium chicken broth
1/2 teaspoon lite salt
2 cups (4 ounces dry weight) bow tie noodles

Place the egg in a bowl and beat lightly. Add kasha and stir until all the kernels are coated. Heat the egg-coated kasha grains in a non-stick pan that has first been coated with 2 teaspoons of the oil, for about 2 to 3 minutes over low heat, or until each grain is separate and dry. Set aside.

Sauté onions in a non-stick skillet in the remaining 2 teaspoons oil. Bring chicken broth to a boil in a medium saucepan. Add the lite salt and sautéed onions. Mix well and add the kasha grains to the broth. Stir for a few seconds, cover, and simmer over low heat for 10 to 15 minutes, or until all the broth is absorbed.

While kasha is simmering in the broth, cook whole grain bow tie noodles according to package directions. Drain noodles and add to the kasha and onions. Mix well and cook gently until thoroughly heated. Serve piping hot.

MILLET PILAF

Serves 4

1 1/4 cups low sodium chicken broth
1/2 cup millet
1/4 cups chopped scallions
Ground black pepper to taste
1/3 cup grated low fat or nonfat mozzarella or Jack cheese
Optional: nonfat sour cream or nonfat yogurt

Bring broth to a boil in a medium saucepan over high heat and add millet. Reduce heat to low and simmer, covered, for 30 to 40 minutes, stirring once or twice. When millet is tender, mix in scallions and pepper to taste and top with grated cheese. Add sour cream or yogurt if desired.

BASIC BARLEY RECIPE

Makes about 8 cups

3 quarts water
1 pound pearl barley, about 2 1/2cups
1/2 teaspoon salt

Combine the water, barley and salt in a large saucepan set over high heat. Bring to a boil, cover, reduce heat and simmer about 20 minutes or until the barley is tender but still crunchy.

Drain well and either cool to room temperature or serve hot.

MORE COMPLEX CARBOHYDRATE RECIPES
STEAMING VEGETABLES

This method is good for many kinds of fresh vegetables: Use a 2 quart saucepan with a tight-fitting lid.[128] Add ½ cup water to the pan, drop in the vegetables, cover, bring to boil over high heat. Then reduce heat to the lowest setting and simmer until the vegetables can be pierced with a fork, but are not soft. You want the finished vegetables to be tender. Serve plain or dusted with Parmesan cheese or garlic or onion powder. In the categories below, begin timing when you turn the heat down to a simmer.

String beans: Cut off ends, cut beans into 1-1/2 inch lengths, cook approximately 7 minutes.

Broccoli: Cut off thick ends, break into florets, cook about 5 minutes.

Cauliflower: Cut florets off central stem. Cook approximately 7 minutes.

Carrots: Cut into ¼ inch rounds. Cook about 3-5 minutes

STIR-FRIED VEGETABLES

Stir-frying is the most versatile technique for cooking vegetables, and the most fun.

[128] Naturally Yours Fat Free Sour Cream has an excellent natural taste that won't be disappointing.

BROCCOLI

The microwave is the working mother's best friend. To make a quick side dish of broccoli, place fresh broccoli florets in a covered bowl with 2 tablespoons of water. Microwave for about 2-3 minutes. Season with squeezed lemon or sprinkle with a small amount of Parmesan cheese.

ASPARAGUS

Young, thin, fresh asparagus is more tender and flavorful. Select only green spears that are about the same length and thickness so they'll all cook at the same rate. Cut away the thick ends, then scrape and wash each spear.

Place one bunch fresh, un-wilted asparagus across the bottom of a large frying pan. Add about one cup of water, cover, bring to a boil, and immediately reduce the heat to a simmer for 1-3 minutes. Don't overcook. As with broccoli, if you overcook asparagus, it loses its dark green color and turns yellow-green.

COLESLAW

Now that you can buy pre-shredded cabbage in the produce section, it's easy to make your own coleslaw and not be held hostage to the store-bought, high-fat type from the delicatessen.

Serves 4

3 tablespoons of your favorite vinegar
3 tablespoons nonfat sour cream[129]
4 teaspoons sugar
1 1/2 cups shredded green cabbage (optional: mix red and green cabbage)
Ground black pepper to taste
Optional: 1/8 teaspoon salt

Combine vinegar, sour cream and sugar in a mixing bowl and stir until smooth. Add the cabbage and toss to coat well. Add pepper, and salt if desired, stirring to combine. Refrigerate at least one hour to enhance flavor. Coleslaw tastes best served cold.

[129] The large green apples are better for baking because they hold their shape better and do not turn into mush.

VEGETABLE SOUP

Soup is a wonderful vegetable delivery system. Here is a basic recipe, but don't be afraid to innovate using your leftover vegetables. For the younger child, use a potato masher on the vegetables once the soup is cooked. As your child adapts to lumpy foods, you can omit this step.

Makes about 10 cups

6 cups low sodium chicken or beef broth
2 carrots, diced
2 whole leeks, diced
1 onion, diced
1 1/2 cups celery, diced
2-3 tablespoons fresh basil, chopped
Pepper to taste—but hold the salt!
Optional: 3 cloves garlic (minced), cauliflower, broccoli, zucchini, summer squash, spinach, tomato, string beans

Combine all ingredients in a large saucepan and bring to a boil. Reduce heat and simmer for 20 minutes. This is your basic preparation, and you may now add any or all of the optional vegetables, cut into small pieces, up to about 2 cups total.

Variation: You may also add cooked white beans, boiled rice, or barley. If adding any of these,reduce some of the basic vegetables so the soup won't be too thick.

VEGETABLE SAUTÉ

Three-year-olds like this sauté, but try it on even younger children. Put it on your plate and see if your child reaches for a taste.

Serves 6

1 yellow onion, chopped
1 clove garlic, sliced
1 sweet red pepper, seeded and cut into 1/4-inch strips
8 medium mushrooms, sliced
2 medium zucchini, sliced 1/8-inch thick
1/4 pound snow pea pods
2 cups cooked brown rice
2 teaspoons Parmesan cheese

Sauté onion in a non-stick pan until soft and slightly browned. Add garlic and red pepper and sauté for 2 minutes. Add mushrooms and zucchini and sauté until zucchini is tender, about 5 minutes, stirring frequently and being careful not to break up the vegetables. Add pea pods and sauté about two more minutes.

Serve over rice, and sprinkle with the Parmesan cheese.

GREEN SALAD WITH VEGETABLES

For children over two years old.

A salad such as the one below used to be time-consuming to prepare, but now ready-cut and washed fresh salad greens come packaged in sealed bags at most supermarkets. Salads such as this should be served daily. The younger child may reject them at first, but make green salad a standard fare.

Serves 4

1/4 head iceberg lettuce
3 to 4 leaves butter lettuce
3 to 4 leaves red leaf lettuce
2 scallions, sliced in 1/4-inch segments (both green and white parts)
1 to 2 stalks celery, sliced into 1/4-inch crescents
1 carrot peeled and sliced into 1/4-inch rounds
2 tablespoons no-sodium garbanzo beans, canned
2 tablespoons no-sodium red kidney beans, canned
Low fat salad dressing

Tear all the lettuce into bite-size pieces. Add the remaining ingredients and toss with low fat dressing.

A nutritious bowl of fresh greens can quickly turn unhealthy when it is smothered in high fat, high salt salad dressing. To avoid this, read labels carefully or prepare your own salad dressing.

HUNGARIAN BUTTER LETTUCE SALAD

Contributed by Mrs. Geri Eszterhas

Serves 4 to 6

2 teaspoons sugar
1 tablespoon white or champagne vinegar
1/4 cup water
1 head butter lettuce
1 large tomato, diced
1 red bell pepper, ribs and seeds removed, diced
1 cucumber, sliced

To make the dressing, dissolve the sugar in vinegar and water and chill.

Wash lettuce, dry well and tear leaves into large pieces. Place lettuce leaves in a salad bowl and add remaining ingredients. Pour all of the dressing over the salad, and toss to combine.

Variation: Another delicious, easy to make, low fat dressing can be prepared by combining 2 tablespoons Dijon mustard, 1 teaspoon honey, and a splash each of lemon and orange juice.

HUNGARIAN CUCUMBERS

Introduce to children over three years old.

Serves 6 to 8

1/4 teaspoon garlic powder
2 tablespoons sugar
3 tablespoons white or champagne vinegar
1/2 cup water
3 large firm cucumbers, peeled and thinly sliced
1 small onion, thinly sliced
1 ripe tomato, cut in wedges
1 bell pepper, ribbing and seeds removed, cut into thin wedges
Sweet Hungarian paprika

To make the dressing, dissolve the garlic powder and sugar in vinegar and water in a salad bowl. Place sliced cucumbers and onion in bowl with the dressing and mix well.

Garnish salad with tomato and bell pepper wedges, and sprinkle the top lightly with paprika.

BAKED POTATO AND BROCCOLI

This vegetable dish can serve as an after school snack or be a part of dinner.

Serves 1 to 2

1 Idaho potato
2 tablespoons nonfat or low fat shredded mozzarella cheese
1 cup steamed broccoli
2 tablespoons fat-free sour cream
2 tablespoons salsa

Bake the potato in the microwave until done, and cut it in half. Top hot potato halves with the cheese, then cover them with broccoli, sour cream and salsa.

CAROL'S BANANA-STRAWBERRY SMOOTHIE

Also good for breakfast on the run. Smoothies are low in fat and appear to be rich in fiber, and they give you at least 2 to 3 servings of fruit.

(The Fiber in a smoothie may lose much of its value. Blending disrupts the fiber of the fruit and vegetables in the process of making the smoothies. It exposes more of the surface area of the food enabling it to be more quickly absorbed. This effects your blood sugar and insulin level and directs the blood sugar to be stored as fat. The blending also makes it easier to consume more calories since there is no need to chew the food. Satiety is delayed. There is a clear difference between the fullness delivered by whole fruit and foods in contrast to the same foods blended. The Smoothie breakfast doesn't have as much "staying power." Therefore, limit smoothies to no more than once a week)

Serves 1

1 cup nonfat milk or nonfat yogurt
1 ripe banana
5 or 6 fresh or frozen strawberries
3 or 4 ice cubes, crushed
1/4 teaspoon vanilla extract
Optional: 1 tablespoon nonfat dry milk (to provide protein, slow digestion, and speed the feeling of satiety).

Process all ingredients in a blender until smooth.

You can find your own perfect smoothie blend through trial and error. Here are some other fruit combinations that make a delicious smoothie:

Four 1-inch chunks of pineapple, and 5 strawberries

- Half a peeled orange, 1 peeled and cored apple
- Half a peeled peach, and 5 strawberries.

BAKED APPLE

This recipe may be increased to make several baked apples.

Serves 1

1 large green baking apple, cored[130]
2 teaspoons apple juice
1 teaspoon brown sugar
1/8 teaspoon cinnamon
Optional: nonfat yogurt or nonfat milk

Preheat oven to 375°F.

Place cored apple in a baking dish.

Combine apple juice, brown sugar, and cinnamon and spoon into the core cavity.

Bake in preheated oven for 45 to 50 minutes, or until the skin turns golden brown and begins to separate from the apple. Serve either warm or cold. Top with nonfat yogurt or cold nonfat milk, if desired.

[130] The tartness of applesauce comes from these crunchy green apples. Choose a sweeter red apple if you prefer a sweet taste and softer texture.

APPLESAUCE

Serves 4

2 to 2 1/2 pounds green apples, slightly tart[131], about 6 medium apples
Enough water to cover apples (about 1/2 cup water)
A few drops lemon juice
Optional: cinnamon and raisins

Peel and core apples and cut into thin wedges. Place in nonstick saucepan with just enough water to cover. (Applesauce will be too thin and watery if excess water is used.)

Add a few drops of lemon juice, cover, and bring to a boil. Reduce heat and simmer for about 10 minutes, stirring occasionally.

When apples become mushy, pour mixture into a blender or food processor. Puree until apples are a fine texture. (A potato masher may be used instead of a blender or food processor.) Add some cinnamon and raisins if desired.

[131] The tartness of applesauce comes from these crunchy green apples. Choose a sweeter red apple if you prefer a sweet taste and softer texture.

PEACH SHERBET

A healthy sweet treat for toddlers and older children.

Serves 4

4 to 5 ice cubes
1 can (16-ounces) yellow cling peach halves (no sugar added), drained, or 4 to 5 fresh ripe peaches in season, coarsely chopped
1/2 cup nonfat milk
1 tablespoon fresh lemon juice
Optional: plain nonfat or reduced fat yogurt

Chop ice cubes in food processor or blender until finely crushed. Add peaches, milk, lemon juice. Blend well.

Pour into ice cube tray and freeze for 1 to 2 hours. Remove several cubes from tray for each serving. Blend frozen cubes until mixture reaches snow cone consistency. Serve in sherbet glasses or small paper cups.

For variety, add some plain nonfat or reduced fat yogurt to frozen peach cubes and blend until mixture becomes slushy.

BAKED PEARS, FRENCH STYLE

These make a convenient lunchbox treat. Chopped up and served on oatmeal or other hot cereal, they will have your child looking forward to a healthy breakfast.

Makes 6 Pear Halves

3 pears, ripe but not soft, halved vertically and cored
1/2 cup water
1 tablespoon sugar
1 teaspoon vanilla extract
1/2 teaspoon cinnamon
Optional: sherbet, plain nonfat yogurt

Preheat oven to 350°F.

Place halved pears, cut side down, in a shallow baking dish. Combine water, sugar, vanilla and cinnamon in a small saucepan and bring to a boil. Reduce heat and simmer, whisking constantly, until sugar is dissolved, about 3 minutes. Pour over pears.

Bake in preheated oven for 15 minutes, until pears are tender when pierced with the tip of a sharp knife.

Serve alone, with sherbet, plain nonfat or reduced fat yogurt.

PROTEIN FOODS RECIPES MEAT, FISH, POULTRY, EGGS, BEANS, TOFU, AND LENTILS

BASIC OMELET

Most children love omelets. They make a great snack, or can be the cornerstone of breakfast, lunch or dinner.

Note: Eggs will be more tender if they're cooked slowly over low heat. This is true for any egg dish, including sunny-side-up eggs.

Makes 1 Omelet

4 egg whites
1 egg yolk (optional)
1/4 cup nonfat milk
Optional: 6 drops Tabasco®
2 teaspoons dehydrated, minced onion flakes
1/4 teaspoon black pepper
Vegetable oil cooking spray
Optional: chili salsa, tomatillo sauce, nonfat or lowfat shredded cheese

Beat eggs with milk until frothy. Add Tabasco if desired. Add onion flakes and pepper. Mix gently. Lightly spray a non-stick skillet with vegetable spray and set it over medium heat.

Pour eggs into heated skillet, cover, and reduce heat to low. Cook for 5 to 7 minutes or until eggs are set.

Variation: After 5 minutes of cooking, add chili salsa, tomatillo sauce, or shredded cheese to the center of the omelet. Fold omelet in half and cook for another 3 to 5 minutes. Pour extra salsa on top just before serving.

LOUIS'S FRENCH TOAST

Makes 2 Slices French Toast

2 egg whites
1 egg yolk
2 tablespoons nonfat milk
2 teaspoons brown sugar
1/2 teaspoon vanilla
1/4 teaspoon cinnamon
2 slices whole wheat bread, preferably slightly stale
Vegetable oil cooking spray

Whisk egg whites, egg yolk, milk, sugar, vanilla and cinnamon in a bowl until well combined. Soak bread in egg mixture until bread is soggy.

Lightly coat a non-stick pan with cooking spray and set over medium-high heat. Fry bread on prepared hot pan until brown on one side. Turn and brown the other side. Serve hot.

SCRAMBLED EGGS WRAPPED IN A TORTILLA

Serves 1

Vegetable oil cooking spray
2 egg whites
1 egg yolk (optional)
1 tablespoon nonfat milk
1 corn or nonfat wheat tortilla
2 tablespoons chili salsa

Lightly coat a non-stick skillet with cooking spray and set over medium heat. Whisk eggs, yolk, and milk together and scramble in prepared pan. In another pan, heat both sides of tortilla until soft,then remove from pan.

Place scrambled eggs in center of tortilla and top with chili salsa. Roll up tortilla and eat while hot.

HUMMUS

Use this garbanzo bean spread as you would use peanut butter. It makes an excellent spread over water crackers, bagels, bread and, for the older child, celery. It also mixes well with tuna.

Makes about 1 ½ Cups

1 can (8 ounces) no-sodium garbanzo beans, drained
3 to 4 drops Tabasco
1/2 clove chopped garlic
1/2 cup low fat or nonfat cottage cheese
1 tablespoon fresh lemon juice
1/4 teaspoon ground coriander

Combine all ingredients in blender or food processor and blend for 30 to 40 seconds, or until smooth.

CHESTNUT STUFFING

Although chestnut stuffing is primarily a recipe enjoyed by older children and adults, it's not too early to introduce this whenever you wish to prepare a stuffing. Many young children adore stuffing, so beginning with a wholesome, low fat one makes nutritional sense.

Makes enough for a 10 to 20 pound turkey or 2 to 3 chickens

1 1/2 pounds chestnuts
1 large apple, peeled, cored and chopped
1 can (8-ounces) water chestnuts, drained
Fresh thyme, to taste
6 celery stalks and leaves, diced
1/2 pound mushrooms, sliced
1/2 cup chopped scallions, white and green parts
4 to 5 cups unseasoned bread crumbs or stale bread (4 slices bread yields about one cup crumbs)

Make crisscross slits over chestnuts and boil in water for 30 minutes. Drain and cool, then remove shells and skins. Remove and discard any moldy or blemished areas.

Place chestnuts in food processor or blender with apple, water chestnuts and thyme and pulse until apple and chestnuts are evenly chopped.

Heat a large non-stick skillet over medium heat and cook celery, mushrooms and scallions until soft. Add chestnut mixture to skillet along with bread crumbs and gently toss to combine. Add enough water to moisten stuffing to desired consistency, mixing with a light hand to keep stuffing from getting heavy.

LENTIL SOUP

Unlike dried beans, lentils do not require soaking and long cooking times. Most toddlers love soups, and this is a great way to introduce vegetables.

Makes about 11 cups, or 6 Servings

1 (16-ounce) package of lentils
2 medium onions, sliced
2 medium carrots, sliced
2 bay leaves
8 cups water
1 cup sliced celery
1/2 teaspoon dried thyme leaves
1/2 teaspoon pepper

Rinse lentils under running cold water and discard any small rocks or shriveled lentils. In a 5–quart Dutch oven or sauce pot, bring lentils and remaining ingredients to a boil over medium heat.

Reduce heat to low, cover, and simmer about 45 minutes or until lentils are tender. Discard bay leaves.

COOKING HINTS FOR PREPARING BEANS

1. A one pound package of dried beans will yield 5-6 cups of cooked beans.
2. A 15 oz. can of beans is equal to about 1-2/3 cups when drained.

To soak beans: In a large bowl or pot combine rinsed beans and enough water to cover by 3-4 inches (about 10 cups of water to a pound of beans.) Let stand at least 8 hours or overnight. Drain the soaking water before proceeding with your recipe.

Quick Soak Method: In a pot, combine rinsed beans with about 10 cups of water to a pound of beans. Bring to a boil and simmer for three minutes. Turn off the heat and set aside for at least an hour. Drain the soaking water before proceeding with your recipe.

BEAN CUISINE'S "THICK AS FOG SPLIT PEA SOUP"

Since there's quite a bit of chopping and mincing in this recipe, I recommend a Cuisinart-type food processor to make life easier.

Serves 8

1 box Bean Cuisine "Thick as Fog Split Pea Soup"[132]
2 tablespoons olive oil
2 cups chopped onions
2 cups chopped celery[133]
2 cups grated carrots
6 cloves garlic, minced
3 cans (16 ounces each) low-sodium, nonfat chicken broth
2 cups water
1/3 pound boneless ham slice, cubed

Remove spice packet from box of soup and reserve 3/4 of the packet for this soup, saving remaining 1/4 packet for another use.

Heat oil in a large pot and sauté onions, celery, carrots and garlic until soft but not browned. Add broth, water, ham, contents of the box and the reserved 3/4 of the spice packet. Bring to a boil, reduce heat and simmer for 2 1/2 to 3 hours, or until peas are soft.

To turn this soup into a tasty and filling lunch, add 1 to 2 tablespoons of cooked rice to each serving bowl.

---

[132] Product of Health House, Reno, Nevada 89509. If not available at your local grocer, contact manufacturer. Also try the "Bag O Beans" soup with chicken!

[133] Celery has a wonderful crunch, has few calories because it is mostly water and, therefore, makes a wonderful low calorie snack for older children. Raw celery should not be given to young children because they can choke on it.

BLACK-EYED PEAS

Use a mild and colorful chili powder in these peas, such as California chili powder. You may also sprinkle the chili powder over eggs, or dust over chicken fillets or shrimp before grilling.

1 pound dried black-eyed peas, soaked overnight or quick soaked (see above)
1 medium onion, chopped
2 ribs celery, chopped
2 bay leaves
8 cups water
2 cups chopped tomatoes
2 teaspoons dried basil
2 teaspoons chili powder[134]
1 teaspoon salt

Combine all ingredients in a large pot. Bring to a boil, cover, reduce heat and simmer for 1 to 1 1/2 hours, stirring occasionally. Serve over rice.

134 Use a mild and colorful chili powder such as California chili powder. Sprinkle chili powder over eggs, dust over chicken fillets or shrimp before grilling.

BEAN DIP

1/2 medium onion, chopped
2 cups cooked black beans
3 to 4 tablespoons fresh chopped cilantro
1 teaspoon ground cumin
1/2 teaspoon salt
1/2 teaspoon ground black pepper

Combine all ingredients in a food processor or blender. Puree until smooth, adding water as necessary to thin to desired consistency.

FRIJOLES (REFRIED BEANS)

Frijoles make an excellent dip with nonfat tortilla chips. Traditionally, they are served with rice on enchilada dishes (see page 212).

2 cups dried pinto beans, washed
2 ounces low fat or nonfat Jack cheese, shredded

Place the washed beans in a large heavy pot with enough water to cover beans by 2 inches (about 4 cups water). Simmer for 3 to 4 hours, or until beans are tender. Add water as necessary to keep beans covered.

When beans are tender, drain and mash them to desired consistency. Fifteen minutes before serving, stir in cheese and reheat if necessary.

PREPARING AND COOKING FISH, MEATS AND POULTRY

Cholesterol varies little regardless of the leanness of a cut of beef, pork, or lamb, but fat content does. The following are some ways to cut down on the fat content of meats, fish and poultry.

Trim all visible fat from meat. Remove all skin from poultry before cooking. Keep in mind that white meat of chicken contains less fat than dark meat. Choose the leanest cuts of meat and avoid steaks that are well marbled. Marbling, remember, is the fat streaks that run through the steak.

Select only extra lean ground meat. If extra lean hamburger is not available, have the butcher grind a well trimmed piece of lean roasting meat such as round. This may actually be less expensive and leaner than the hamburger on the display counter at your supermarket. When buying canned tuna, select only the "reduced sodium" water packed tuna. Avoid the oil packed or regular water packed tuna.

When a recipe calls for browning, frying, or saute'ing, brown under the broiler. Broil or bake meats or poultry on a rack to drain off fat. Drain hamburgers or other meats further by patting with a paper towel. Discard any fat after cooking. This significantly decreases the fat content of your food.

Or saute' with water, a mixture of lemon juice and water or garlic juice and water on a non-stick pan. Take care to use a plastic spatula to prevent damage to the non-stick surface.

Fish should be broiled, baked or poached, not fried. Breaded fish can be browned under the broiler to simulate frying, but avoid Shake'n Bake type of products because of their extremely high fat content. Do not overcook fish. Avoid covering meat or fish with fatty, rich sauces.

Finally, it I a good idea to eat smaller portions that you are used to of the meats highest in fat such as beef, pork, and lamb. Your will begin to find yourself no longer desiring the large quantities of meat found in many American diets.

"FRIED" FILLET OF FISH

If you want to thaw frozen fish, place it in the refrigerator. Do not thaw it at room temperature where it may be subject to bacterial contamination. If you wish to cook fish while it is still frozen, double the cooking time, but for this recipe allow the fish to thaw.

Serves 4

1 pound white fish (fillet of any firm white-fleshed fish such as orange roughy, cod, haddock, or halibut)
1 tablespoon plain nonfat yogurt
1 tablespoon Dijon-style mustard
1 tablespoon chopped chives
1 tablespoon chopped parsley
California chili powder or any mild chili powder to taste
1 1/2 cups corn flakes, crushed
Vegetable oil cooking spray
Preheat oven to 375°F.

Rinse the fish quickly with cold water and pat dry. Run your finger across each fillet to check for bones. If you feel the tips of any bones, pull them out with a tweezers.

Cut the fish in four equal pieces. Combine yogurt, mustard, chives, parsley and chili powder (or pepper). Rub mixture onto all sides of fish and marinate in refrigerator for 15 to 20 minutes.

Coat fish on all sides with generous amounts of crushed corn flakes. Spray a baking sheet with the vegetable oil spray and place fish on the baking sheet so the fillets are separated from each other.

Bake in preheated oven for 10 minutes, or until done.

To test fish for doneness, use a fork or the tip of a knife to see if fish flakes easily. The fish should barely flake, and be just opaque and no longer translucent. The fish will continue to cook from retained heat even after it is removed from the oven, so it may be best to stop cooking it when fish is just a shade underdone.

*Ground red pepper may be substituted, but use sparingly.

RED SNAPPER VERACRUZANA

Enjoyed even by children who do not like fish!

Serves 4

Sauce Veracruzana (see page)
1 pound red snapper or rock fish
Fresh cilantro, chopped

Prepare Veracruzana sauce as directed.

Preheat broiler for about 5 minutes. Place fish fillets on Teflon or non-stick broiler pan or baking sheet. Broil fish for approximately 5 minutes without turning.

The fish should barely flake, be just opaque, and no longer translucent. (Better to undercook slightly than to overcook. Over-cooking fish markedly decreases its flavor.)

With the aid of a pancake turner, carefully slide fish to a heated platter. Pour warm Veracruzana sauce over the fish. Sprinkle with chopped cilantro and serve immediately.

BEAN AND TURKEY DINNER

When children grow up eating dishes based on beans and vegetables, they will keep these good habits as adults.

Serves 4 to 6

1/2 pound ground turkey
1 onion, chopped
1 garlic clove, chopped
1 1/2 cups dry macaroni
2 1/2 cups low-sodium broth or water
1 can (15-ounces) low-sodium kidney beans, drained
1 cup chopped ripe tomatoes
1 1/2 teaspoons dried oregano
1 teaspoon chili powder
1/4 teaspoon salt
1/4 teaspoon ground black pepper
1/4 cup grated mozzarella cheese

Brown ground turkey in a large non-stick skillet. When turkey is barely cooked, add onion and garlic and cook until onion is translucent but not browned. Turn heat to low and mix in macaroni, broth or water, beans, tomatoes and seasonings.

Cover and simmer about 20 minutes, or until macaroni is tender, stirring occasionally. Remove from heat and sprinkle with grated cheese. Cover and let the cheese melt.

LOW-FAT TURKEY GRAVY

Collect drippings from a roasted turkey, including the brown solids on the bottom of the pan. To de-fat drippings, allow them to set until the fat rises (place in the freezer for quicker results). Remove the clear broth with a bulb baster, or spoon fat off if drippings have been placed in freezer and become solid.

Makes about 2 ¾ cups

2 1/2 cups defatted turkey broth (supplement with low sodium canned chicken broth)
1/4 cup all-purpose flour
1/4 cup cold water

Combine defatted turkey broth and canned broth (to equal 2 1/2 cups total) in a skillet and bring to a simmer.

Whisk the flour and cold water in a bowl until well combined. Slowly add flour mixture to the simmering broth, whisking constantly until the gravy thickens.

You may add a small amount of seasoning such as Molly McButter or Lite Salt. My wife adds some Tabasco or Worcestershire sauce to the gravy to enhance its taste, but not too much because of the salt content.

TURKEY MEATBALLS

Meatballs go well with pasta, or sliced in a sandwich. Use a sourdough or French roll for a traditional meatball sandwich. Toppings such as pizza sauce, salsa, or melted nonfat shredded mozzarella make meatball sandwiches a favorite.

Serves 2

8 ounces ground turkey breast
2 egg whites, beaten
1 1/2 tablespoons ketchup
Vegetable oil cooking spray

Preheat oven to 375°F.

Combine all ingredients in a large mixing bowl. Roll into small meatballs about one inch in diameter.

Place meatballs on a non-stick baking sheet that has been coated with cooking spray. Bake in preheated oven for about 20 minutes, or until meatballs are cooked through and lightly browned.

KIM'S CHICKEN IN ORANGE SAUCE

The sweeter the orange juice, the better the results in this recipe.

Serves 4

4 chicken breast halves, boned and skinned
1 cup all-purpose flour
3/4 cup fresh orange juice
1/3 cup Chablis or other white wine
1/3 cup slice fresh mushrooms
2 tablespoons finely chopped fresh parsley
1 teaspoon orange zest
1 pinch dried rosemary
2 tablespoons raspberry or champagne vinegar
Garnish: fresh, peeled and pitted orange slices

Pound or cut chicken breast halves to an even thickness. Coat chicken pieces lightly in flour, shaking off excess flour.

Sauté chicken (without oil) in a non-stick skillet. Brown well on both sides.

Add orange juice, Chablis, mushrooms, parsley, orange zest and rosemary to skillet and bring to a simmer. Cover and simmer for 7 minutes.

Transfer chicken to a heated serving platter and cover with foil to keep warm. Add vinegar to skillet and bring to a simmer again, simmering until sauce is reduced by one-third, stirring frequently. Pour sauce over chicken and garnish with orange slices.

All CARMINE'S recipes were contributed by the late Chef Michael Ronis of CARMINE'S Restaurant, 200 West 44th Street, New York, NY 10036; Telephone: (212) 221-3800.

CARMINE'S BARBECUED CHICKEN

Each serving contains approximately 135 calories.

Serves 8

8 chicken legs
Garlic powder to taste
2 cups barbeque sauce

Preheat oven to 350°F.

Place the chicken legs in a baking dish and sprinkle lightly with garlic powder. Cover the baking dish with a lid or aluminum foil and bake in preheated oven for 30 minutes.

Remove chicken from oven and allow to cool until the legs can be handled easily.

Remove and discard chicken skin and place legs back in the dish, pouring off any fat.

Pour 1/4 cup of the sauce over each chicken leg. Cover and bake for 20 minutes longer.

CARMINE'S CHICKEN CACCIATORE

An alternate way to serve this dish would be to chop the cooked chicken, add to cooked pasta and top with the sauce. Each serving contains approximately 125 calories.

Serves 8

3 tomatoes, peeled and diced
2 large onions, finely chopped
2 cloves garlic, finely chopped
1 tablespoon dried rosemary, crushed using a mortar and pestle
2 teaspoons dried oregano, crushed using a mortar and pestle
1 1/2 teaspoons olive oil
4 whole chicken breasts, boned, skinned and cut into halves
Salt
Freshly ground black pepper
1 cup dry Marsala wine
1 cup dry white wine
1 can (6-ounces) tomato paste

Combine the tomatoes, onions, garlic, rosemary and oregano and mix well. Spread the mixture evenly over the bottom of a baking dish.

Heat the oil in a large skillet. Lightly sprinkle both sides of the chicken breasts with salt and pepper. Place chicken in the skillet and brown evenly on both sides.

Arrange the chicken on top of the tomato-onion mixture in the baking dish and bake, covered, in preheated oven for 10 minutes.

Combine the Marsala, white wine and tomato paste and mix well. Pour over the tops of the chicken breast halves and bake, covered, 20 minutes longer.

To serve, place each chicken breast half on a plate. Mix the sauce in the baking dish to a smooth texture and spoon over the chicken.

CARMINE'S CRUSTLESS CHICKEN PIZZA

Each serving contains approximately 190 calories.

Serves 8

Sauce
1 large onion, finely chopped
2 cloves garlic, finely chopped
2 cups tomato sauce
1 1/2 teaspoons dried oregano, crushed using a mortar and pestle
1/2 teaspoon freshly ground black pepper
1/4 teaspoon salt

1 1/2 teaspoons olive oil
4 whole chicken breasts, boned, skinned and cut into halves
1 cup grated part skim mozzarella cheese

Preheat oven to 400°F.

Combine the onion and garlic in a medium saucepan and cook, covered, over very low heat until soft, stirring frequently to prevent scorching. Add remaining sauce ingredients and bring to a boil. Reduce heat and simmer, uncovered, for 1 hour, stirring occasionally.

While sauce is simmering, heat oil in a large skillet and cook chicken breasts until they are lightly browned on both sides.

Arrange the chicken breast halves in a baking dish and spoon the sauce evenly over the tops. Sprinkle 2 tablespoons of the cheese over each "chicken pizza." Bake, uncovered, in preheated oven for about 20 minutes, until chicken is no longer pink in the center and the cheese is melted and lightly browned.

CARMINE'S CHICKEN ENCHILADAS

Each serving contains approximately 230 calories.

Serves 8

3 onions, finely chopped
2 cloves garlic, finely chopped
2 tablespoons chili powder
1 teaspoon salt
1 teaspoon ground cumin
1 can (28-ounces) sodium-free tomatoes, undrained
2 cups diced cooked chicken
1 cup grated reduced-fat sharp cheddar cheese, divided
8 corn tortillas, warmed

Preheat oven to 350°F.

Combine onion and garlic in a large non-stick saucepan and cook, covered, over very low heat until soft, stirring frequently to prevent scorching.

Add the chili powder, salt and cumin to the pan and mix well. Pour the juice from the can of tomatoes into the pan. Chop the tomatoes and add to sauce.

Continue to cook, covered, for 10 minutes. Pour half the sauce into a bowl and reserve. Add the chicken and 1/2 cup of the grated cheese to the remaining sauce in the pan and mix well.

Spoon 1/8 of the mixture from the pan in the center of each tortilla and roll the tortilla around filling. Place the enchiladas, seam side down, in a baking dish. Spoon the reserved sauce evenly over the tops of the enchiladas and sprinkle 1 tablespoon of the remaining grated cheese over each enchilada. Bake, covered, in preheated oven for 30 minutes.

VANDA'S SPAGHETTI PIE

(Recipe contributed by Vanda Braun)

Serves 4 to 6

6 ounces (uncooked weight) spaghetti, cooked al dente and drained
1/4 cup grated low fat or nonfat mozzarella cheese
1 whole egg, beaten
1 egg white, beaten
Meat Sauce
1 pound ground round, extra lean
1/2 cup chopped green pepper
1 medium onion, chopped
1 can (8-ounces) sodium-free stewed tomatoes
1 can (3-ounces) sodium-free tomato paste
2 teaspoons garlic powder
1 teaspoon oregano
1 cup low-fat or nonfat cottage cheese
1/3 cup grated low fat or nonfat mozzarella cheese, additional

Preheat oven to 350°F.

Place hot, drained spaghetti in a bowl, add the ¼ cup mozzarella and mix well. Allow spaghetti-cheese mixture to cool for a few minutes, and then stir in beaten egg and white. Spread into a 10-inch non-stick or glass pie pan and form spaghetti into a bottom crust.

Meat Sauce:

Prepare sauce by browning ground meat in a large skillet over medium heat. When meat releases some juices, add green pepper and onion and cook over medium heat until meat is browned and vegetables are softened, 10 to 15 minutes. Add stewed tomatoes, tomato paste, garlic powder and oregano to meat in skillet and mix to thoroughly combine.

Spread cottage cheese evenly over spaghetti "crust" in the 10-inch pan, and top with the meat sauce. Bake in preheated oven for 20 to 30 minutes. Remove from oven and sprinkle additional mozzarella on top. Return to oven and bake for 5 minutes, or until cheese melts.

BEAN BURRITO

Serves 1

Recipe may be increased to make as many burritos as you want.

For each burrito:

2 1/2 tablespoons fat-free refried beans
1 corn or nonfat whole wheat tortilla
1 tablespoon shredded nonfat mozzarella cheese
2 tablespoons fat-free sour cream
2 tablespoons fresh salsa

Heat 2 1/2 tablespoons refried beans in microwave until hot. Spread the hot beans in the center of a tortilla. Sprinkle the shredded cheese over the beans. Place the tortilla with the beans and cheese in the microwave for 20 seconds or until the cheese is soft.

Remove tortilla from the microwave, and add the sour cream and salsa. Fold one end of the tortilla and wrap it as a blinz or crepe.

CHICKEN OR TURKEY ENCHILADAS

Leftover enchiladas can be frozen and reheated to make a quick lunch or after school snack.

Serves 6

6 corn tortillas or nonfat wheat tortillas
2 1/2 cups shredded broiled or baked skinless chicken or turkey breast
8 ounces reduced-sodium chile salsa
Optional: 1 can (4 ounces) diced green chiles
8 ounces reduced-sodium tomatillo sauce
6 ounces shredded low fat Swiss, or low fat or nonfat Monterey Jack cheese
Suggested accompaniments: Low fat or nonfat refried beans and Spanish rice.

Preheat oven to 350°F.

To prepare corn tortillas so they won't crack when rolled: wrap them in a damp kitchen towel, wrap towel in foil and place in preheated oven for about 10 minutes. This will soften the tortillas. This can also be done more quickly in the microwave, without the foil.

Mix shredded chicken or turkey with chile salsa (and canned green chiles, if desired) in a large saucepan and simmer, covered, for about 15 minutes. Place about 1/3 cup of the mixture in the center of each tortilla.

Roll up the tortillas and place, seam side down, in a non-stick baking dish. Pour tomatillo sauce over tortillas and sprinkle with cheese. Bake in preheated oven for about 15 minutes, or until the cheese melts.

Serve on heated dishes with low fat or nonfat refried beans (frijoles) and Spanish Rice.

CREAMY POTATO SOUP

Creamy Potato Soup Mix is a product of Bear Creek Country Kitchens, 325 W. 600 S. Heber City, UT, 84032. Questions or comments call 800-516-7286.

This soup can be prepared in a jiffy and is low in salt and fat. It may be the vehicle to deliver your toddler a variety of vegetables. Chopped up clams and white fish turn this soup into a chowder.

2 cups water
2/3 cup Creamy Potato Soup Mix
Additions: peas, broccoli, corn, leftover vegetables, bay shrimp[135]
Ground black pepper to taste
Small amount of salt

Bring water to a boil in a medium saucepan. Add soup mix to boiling water and simmer 15 to 20 minutes. Add any of the above additions and simmer for another 15 to 20 minutes. Add pepper and a small amount of salt.

The vegetables add the needed fiber and other important nutrients to the soup.

[135] Avoid shrimp or clams if there is a strong family history of food allergy or eczema.

MEDITERRANEAN BLACK BEAN SOUP

This recipe is included to illustrate how easy it is to convert a high-salt, prepared mix into a delicious, wholesome, low fat, high-fiber, reduced sodium meal.

MANISCHEWITZ HOMESTYLE SOUP MIX

The label reads: "With Manischewitz Homestyle Soup Mix, you can make nutritious entrees (in just one pot) that your whole family will love! We have combined a carefully selected blend of beans with savory herbs and rice to help you create a delicious homemade soup."

Here is the original recipe as it appears on the box:
1 box Manischewitz Homestyle Mediterranean Bean Soup
1 onion, chopped
7 cups water
1 15-oz can chopped tomatoes or tomato sauce
1 cup celery, chopped
salt and pepper to taste

In large pot, add water, bean package, onion, tomatoes and celery. Bring to a boil reduce heat, cover and simmer 1 1/2 hours or until beans are tender. Stir occasionally. Add seasoning and rice packet and continue simmering for 1/2 hour. Serve topped with chopped scallions or a dollop of sour cream. Makes six 1 cup servings.

If meat is desired: brown 1/2 - 1 lb. ground beef or other meat choice and add to soup for last 1/2 hour of cooking.

Now here is how you modify the recipe and make it truly nutritious:

Makes 6 one cup servings.

6 cups water (instead of 7 cups)
1 box Manischewitz Homestyle Mediterranean Bean Soup
1 onion, chopped
1 can (15-ounces) sodium-free stewed tomatoes (instead of chopped tomatoes or tomato sauce)
1 cup celery, hopped
1 cup sliced carrots (added to recipe)
1 1/2 cups cooked rice
A pinch of red pepper flakes (instead of salt and pepper to taste)

Chopped scallions for garnish

In a large pot place water, box of bean soup, onion, tomatoes, celery, and carrots. Bring to a boil, reduce heat, cover and simmer 1 1/2 hours or until beans are tender, stirring occasionally.

Add 1/3 of the seasoning packet in the box instead of the whole packet, the rice and the pepper flakes. Continue simmering for 1/2 hour. Serve topped with chopped scallions, but skip the dollop of sour cream (as suggested in the recipe on the box).

If meat is desired: Brown 1/2 to 1 pound extra lean ground beef or ground turkey and add to soup for last 1/2 hour of cooking.

The food industry doesn't spend billions of advertising dollars to promote good food choices. They are bombarding your children with food and candy advertisements during the TV cartoon hours, thus shaping poor food preferences. As a parent you must take responsibility for what you and your children eat. To help you do that, video tape your child's favorite TV programs and delete the advertisements. Keep a library of videotapes. Kids love re-runs. This is the first proactive step needed to capture or re-capture your child's mind. Nutrition goes well beyond the belly!

Become active in your PTA and School Lunch Program. Have other members of your group read this book and they will learn why truly good nutrition is one of the most important gifts a parent can give a child. The common sense of your concerns and recommendations will become clear. You will win allies to promote healthier foods in school and at after school activities.

Parents must become more involved in the food selections made for our children. Insist and demand that the lunches served in school should be the gold standard or model for optimal nutrition. Give a copy of this book to any member of your community who is involved in making these far reaching decisions. Habits begin at an early age, and we as adults all know how difficult it is to make changes in food choices. Your efforts will go a long way to eliminate those diseases of advancing age that we needlessly endure. They need not be inevitable. Our next generation of adults should not have their quality of life sacrificed by eating habits that lead to obesity, early heart disease, colon and prostate cancer, gallbladder disease, diverticulosis, diabetes and stroke.

FAST FOODS

▲ ▲ ▲

Let's face it. Your children are going to be eating "fast foods," and you probably will join in. As I said earlier, this isn't a perfect world, and to survive, compromise must be part of your menu. This section is not for those readers who believe they have total control of their children's diets and never eat at fast food joints. However, you still might enjoy reading about how us weak ones deal with the pressures to eat high fat, high sodium, low fiber inexpensive foods.

THESE NUTRITIONAL FACTS ARE INCLUDED TO HELP YOU BECOME A MORE INFORMED CONSUMER

The next time you are at the airport waiting for your delayed flight, consider these food facts before selecting a mega-dose of fat, sodium and sugar. Check the calories and other Nutrition Facts now listed on the menu!

McDonald's

Best Choice: Hamburger is about 260 calories with 9 grams fat. Compare with other menu items.

Burger King

Broiler Chicken (without mayo) is 370 calories and 9 grams of fat. Check menu to see whether they offer a better choice.

Hardee's: Sub-contains 370 calories and 5 grams of fat. Hamburger is 260 calories with 10 grams of fat, but Pancakes are 280 calories with only 2 grams of fat. But behold the sugar.

Taco Bell

Menus keep changing, but select the best of the worst. How does Pintos n' Cheese sound? 190 calories plus 9 grams of fat.

Pizza Hut:

Veggie Pizza (2 slices) provides 380 calories that includes 16 grams of fat.

Subway

This fast food chain boasts of, "7 subs with 6 grams of fat or less." This is true if you don't add mayo and cheese. But check out the sodium. The turkey breast sub has over 1400mg! So if this is your selection, please don't make it worse by adding pickles.

Arby's:

How does Light Roast Turkey sound with 260 calories including 6 grams of fat?

III. NUTRITIONAL FACTS READING FOOD LABELS

(LEAVE SPACE FOR A NUTRITIONAL FACTS LABEL)

Now that you are fortified with a strong understanding of nutrition, it's time to go shopping and make intelligent food choices. The food label may help you, but only if you understand the special vocabulary used, and the little deceptive tricks employed by those who want you to buy their products. Once understood, you will become a skillful shopper. To be able to see through the hype and half-truths of a sales pitch is an empowerment that gives both strength and joy to any consumer.

DEFINITIONS

Serving size - the serving size is the first bit of information listed under the NUTRITION FACTS label. This amount is set by the FDA and not the manufacturer. Serving size is often an idealized amount rather than what you or most people would eat.

Percent Daily Values (DV) are based on a 2000 calorie diet. This is of little value for the parent looking for guidelines for their child or adolescent who may consume fewer or more than 2000 calories per day. Even so, the acceptable amount of fat listed is excessive. Total fat should be 45 grams or less for those consuming a 2000 calorie diet. For teenagers consuming a 2500 calorie diet, total fat should be kept below 55 grams. Children consuming 1500 calories a day should limit their fat to 35 grams or less.

Low-Fat - No more than three grams of fat per serving of an individual food. The labeling law is different for a box that contains a whole meal.

If a main dish or whole meal is labeled "low fat" it means that it contains no more than 30% of its calories from fat, and that is not low fat! Keep in mind that 30% is listed as a maximum! In the real world most consumers turn the maximum into the minimum. A truly low fat meal is one that is no more than 20% of calories from fat. **The decision to use 30% to represent low-fat was a political one and not based on our present nutritional knowledge. Almost all nutritional studies have demonstrated that the heart benefits of a reduced fat diet ARE NOT DEMONSTRATED AT 30% CALORIES FROM FAT! The studies DO show that a 20% calories from fat or less DOES decrease cardiovascular disease. A diet containing 20%-25% calories from fat is not extremely low fat has been shown not to be harmful to the growth and development of young children or adolescents[136].**

Low in saturated fat: No more than one gram of saturated fat per individual serving or less than 10% of calories from saturated fat in a meal or main dish.

Light or "Lite": The fat content or calories must be cut in half. The label should tell which one. Light can also mean one half the usual sodium content.

Lean: The USDA defines lean as less than 10 grams of fat in the meal; less than 4 grams of saturated fat, and less than 95 mg of cholesterol. (per 100 grams or 3-1/2 ounces)

Extra – Lean[137]: Less than 5 grams of fat in a meal or main dish; less than 2 grams of saturated fat, and less than 95 mg of cholesterol. (per 100 grams or 3-1/2 ounces)

---

136 Pediatr 1998;133:28-34.

137 Labels are sometimes confusing (deceptive?). For example: **Extra-lean**

For meals and main dishes, look for no more than 2 grams of fat and less than 1 gram of saturated fat for every 100 calories. Thus a 250 calorie meal should contain no more than 5 grams of fat and less than 2-1/2 grams of saturated fat.

Cholesterol Free: Less than 2 mg of cholesterol and no more than 2 mg of saturated fat per serving.

Good source: Must contain at least 10% of the Daily Value of the nutrient.
High source: Must contain at least 20% of the Daily Value of the nutrient.
Good source or High source could be used deceptively by suggesting this is a healthy food. For example, if a meal contains a vegetable such as broccoli, the package may claim "Contains broccoli, a good source of folic acid" but have a high fat or salt content.

Calories: The total calories per serving.
Calorie - free: Fewer than 5 calories per serving
Low Calorie: 40 calories or less per serving (and per 50 grams of food).
Reduced Calories: A product altered to contain 25 percent fewer calories than the comparable food without reduced calories.

Calories from fat: The calories from fat, which you wish to keep low. One gram of fat is equal to 9 calories. If Total Fat on the nutrition label is 10 grams, then the calories from fat is (9 X 10) 90 calories.

Unless you're a mathematician this figure won't help the typical shopper too much. Instead the label should contain the value of **percent calories from fat.** That would rapidly give some

---

ground beef contains 16 grams of fat per 100 grams or 3-1/2 ounces. Refer to earlier section comparing beef cuts.

much needed nutritional information. The percent of calories from fat should ideally be no more than 20-25%.

Total Carbohydrate: This part of the label does not offer too much information because it does not separate complex carbohydrate from simple carbohydrates (sugar).

Sugars: The amount of naturally occurring as well as added sugars; omits some of the other sugars such as corn syrup. The amount of sugar, therefore, can be a larger amount than stated.
Sugar Free: Less than 1/2 gram per serving.
Sodium: Try to keep the milligrams of sodium to as much as or less than the **Calories** on the Nutrition Facts label. That is, if there are 100 calories per serving, the milligrams of sodium should be 100 mg or less per serving. Try to avoid prepared meals that contain more than 450 mg of sodium per serving.

2000 calorie diet should contain less than 2000 mg of sodium.
1500 calorie diet should contain less than 1500 mg of sodium
1000 calorie diet should contain less than 1000 mg of sodium

Sodium Free: Less than 5 mg per serving
Low Sodium: Less than 140 mg per serving and per 50 grams of food.
Very Low Sodium: Less than 35 mg per serving and per 50 grams of food.
Sodium, Lite or Light: If the sodium content of a low-calorie, low-fat food has been reduced by half.

Fresh Frozen: freshly frozen, frozen fresh. (A conflict of meanings!)
A Source of: One serving must contain at least 10-19 percent of the adult daily requirement of the named nutrient.

Reduced or Less: Contains at least 25 percent less of the named substance than the food usually contains.

More: One serving contains at least 10 percent more of the Daily Value (DV) than the food it is being compared with.

Ingredients: Ingredients are listed by weight, from the most to the least. If corn syrup, molasses, sugar, maltose, fructose are high on the list, the food probably is loaded with simple sugars. When oil, butter, hydrogenated fats or oils, cheese, or lard are represented high on the list, the food may have excessive amounts of saturated fats and cholesterol. When the ingredients label says, "May contain one or more of the following: soybean oil and /or palm oil," it means either one may be substituted for the other. (Usually depending upon which one is less expensive or more available at the moment). Look for the words, salt, sodium, soy sauce, sodium bicarbonate, seaweed, and sea salt as indicators that you are dealing with a high salt food.

The most important thing to remember is that the ingredients are listed in descending order of predominance. The first two or three ingredients are the ones that matter most.

MAKING FOOD CHOICES: USING THE NEW FOOD LABEL

To gather the most practical information from the Nutrition Facts and Ingredients labels, approach each food with a few basic questions.

1. How many grams of saturated fat are present per serving? Try to keep it **below** 2 grams per serving. If this is not possible, compare products and select the one with the least fat.
2. Next, look for the sodium content per serving. Use the rule of thumb: one gram of sodium for each calorie per

serving. This may be difficult when buying cheese, pizza, soup and other intrinsically high sodium foods. Here, the compromise rule may be expanded to read: 2 grams of sodium for each calorie per serving. Check different brands and select the one with the least sodium.

3. The fiber content of the food is the next important issue. If fiber is not listed, it means there is no significant fiber in the product. When choosing a cereal for your child (or for yourself) look for one that has 3 grams or more of fiber per serving (but not too high in sodium, saturated fat, or simple sugar).
   The word, "Whole" as in Whole Grains should appear as the first or second listed whether whole wheat, oats, rye, or another grain.

4. Check the Nutrition Facts and Ingredients labels for the amount of simple sugar. Avoid cereal products that say, "Frosted" and be careful when the label reads, "lightly sweetened." Select cereals that contain no more than 4 grams of **added sugar** per serving. **Remember that juice is 100% sugar and water. The container may say no sugar added, but that does not mean it is without sugar. Fruit "drinks" and sodas should be avoided. Instead choose beverages such as water, herbal or green tea.**

5. Finally check for vitamin and mineral content. Specifically look for Vitamin C, Folic Acid, Calcium and Iron.

THE 10 WORST FOODS ACCORDING TO THE CENTER FOR SCIENCE IN THE PUBLIC INTEREST-2012

1. Marie Callender's Chicken Pot Pie: Why? Because one serving contains 520 calories; 11 grams of saturated fat; 800 mg of sodium; and if you eat the entire pie as most people do-you will consume 1040 calories of which 22 grams are of saturated fat and 1600 mg of sodium.
2. Olive Garden's Tour of Italy: Why? Because it comes with Lasagna, Breaded Chicken Parmigiana, and Creamy Fettuccine Alfredo and contains 1450 calories; 33 grams of saturated fat; and 3830 grams of sodium. And it comes with a plate of Garden-Fresh Salad with dressing that contains an additional 350 calories and 1930 mg of sodium!!
3. Campbell's Chicken Noodle Soup: One cup of Campbell's Condensed soup has 760mg sodium
4. Chipotle Chicken Burrito: Why? Because it has 970 calories; 18 grams of saturated fat; and 2200 mg sodium. Most teens eat two!!
5. The Cheesecake Factory's Chocolate Tower Truffle Cake: Why? 1679 calories and 49 grams fat.
6. Pillsbury Grands! Cinnabon Roll with icing: Why? 310 calories and 2 grams of saturated fat plus 2.5 grams of trans fat-from partially hydrogenated oils; 5 teaspoons of sugar. Do you need more reasons?
7. Land O'Lakes Margarine: Why? Because each teaspoon of the spread has 11 grams total fat of which 3 grams are saturated fat. This plus partially hydrogenated soybean oil and cottonseed oil. ?hidden trans-fats?

8. **Starbucks Venti White Chocolate Mocha with 2% milk and whipped cream: Why? Because it has 550 calories and 15 grams of saturated fat. This is worse than McDonald Quarter Pounder with Cheese.**

9. **Haagen-Daz ice cream: Why? Because a petite half-cup contains 260 calories and 17 grams of fat plus 21 grams (over 5 teaspoons) sugar. And what teenager eats only a ½ cup?**

10. **Cold Stone Creamery's Oh Fudge shake (large): Why? Because it dumps 1750, calories loaded with 118 grams of fat-64 grams are saturated, plus 140 grams (29-1/2 teaspoons) of sugar into your stomach without killing your appetite. This is the fat and calorie equivalent 2 pounds of T-Bone steak and a buttered baked potato.**

10 MORE WORST FOODS

CARL'S JR. SIX DOLLAR GUACAMOLE BACON BURGER WITH MEDIUM NATURAL CUT FRIES AND 32 oz COKE: 1750 calories, 93 grams of fat, 1.5 trans fat, 3175 mg sodium.

Outback Steakhouse Baby Back Ribs:1539 calories, 96 grams of fat or which 38 grams are saturated and 1675 mg sodium.

Worst Pizza: Uno Chicago Grill Classic Deep Dish Individual Pizza: 2310 calories, 165 grams total fat with 54 grams being saturated, and 4650 grams of sodium. WOW!!

Baja Fresh Charbroiled Steak Nachos: 2120 calories, 118 total fat with 44 grams being saturated, 4.5 grams trans fat, and 2990 mg sodium.

Applebee's New England Fish & Chips: 1930 calories, 138 total fat with 24 grams saturated and 1.5 grams trans fat, 3180 mg sodium.

P.F. Chang's Combo Double Pan-Fried Noodles: 1820 calories, 84 grams total fat with 8 grams saturated, 7692 mg sodium.

IHOP's Big Steak Omelette: 1210 calories, 81 grams total fat with 27 grams saturated and 1.5 trans fat, 2389 mg sodium.

Worst Frozen Breakfast: Jimmy Dean Pancake and Sausage Breakfast Bowl: 710 calories, 34 grams total fat with 12 grams saturated, 1000 mg sodium and 35 grams sugar.

Worst Supermarket Kids' Lunch: Oscar Mayer Deep Dish Pizza with Pepperoni Lunchables: 500 calories, 22 grams total fat of which 8 grams are saturated and .5 grams are trans fats, 890 mg sodium, 28 grams (7 teaspoons) sugar.

Worst Canned Fruit: Del Monte Peach Chunks Yellow Cling Peaches in Heavy Syrup: 100 calories and 23 grams of sugar (6 teaspoons).

READING NUTRITION FACTS FOOD LABELS

▲ ▲ ▲

BREAKFAST FOODS

ONE PLANET TOTALLY FREE ORGANIC GRANOLA

Mulberries, Blueberries, Coconut, Pumpkin Seeds

Gluten Free & Vegan

Nutrition Facts	
Calories	230
Calories From Fat	70
Total Fat	8 grams
Saturated Fat	2 grams
Cholesterol	0
Sodium	10 mg
Total Carbohydrate	34 grams
Dietary Fiber	5 grams
Sugars	7 grams
Protein	7 grams

OAT MEAL

Oatmeal is a great source of fiber. The slow cooking oatmeal (about 15-20 minutes) has 6 grams of fiber compared to the 3 grams found in the instant type.

QUAKER INSTANT OATMEAL
with real apple and cinnamon

Nutrition Facts
Serving Size 1 packet

Calories 130	
	Calories from Fat 15
Total Fat 1.5 grams	
	Saturated Fat 0.5 grams
Cholesterol 0 mg	
Sodium 120 mg	
Total Carbohydrate 27 grams	
	Dietary Fiber 3 grams
	Soluble Fiber 1 gram
	Sugars 11 grams How many grams of sugar are added?
	There is know way of telling from the Nutrition Label.
Protein 3 grams	

QUAKER OATS
(OLD FASHIONED)

Nutrition Facts
Serving Size _ cup
Servings Per Container 13

Amount Per Serving About
Calories 150
Calories from Fat 25
Total Fat 3 grams
Saturated Fat 0.5 grams
Polyunsaturated Fat 1 gram
Monounsaturated Fat 1 gram
Cholesterol 0 mg
Sodium 0 mg
Total Carbohydrate 27grams
Dietary Fiber 4 grams
Soluble Fiber 2 grams
Insoluble Fiber 2 grams
Sugars 1 gram
Protein 5 grams
Vitamin A 0% **Vitamin C** 0%
Calcium 0% **Iron** 10%

CHEERIOS[135]
TOASTED WHOLE GRAIN OAT CEREAL

Nutrition Facts
Serving Size: 1 CUP
Servings Per Container: 14
Amount Per Serving
Calories: 110
Calories from Fat 15
Total Fat 2 grams
Saturated Fat 0.5 grams
Cholesterol 0 g
Sodium 280 mg
Potassium 95 mg
Total Carbohydrate 22 grams
Dietary Fiber 3 grams
soluble fiber 1 gram
insoluble fiber 2 grams
Sugars 1 gram ___(1/4 teaspoon)___
other carbohydrate 18 grams
Protein 3 grams __________
Thiamin % **Riboflavin** % **Niacin** % **Iron** % **Calcium** %

[138] Amount in cereal. One half cup skim milk contributes an additional 40 calories, 65 mg sodium,

200 mg potassium, 6 grams total carbohydrate (6 grams sugars) and 4 grams protein.

Let's compare cereals.
It may be time to change what you're buying your child.

FROSTED CHEERIOS
"LOW FAT" and VERY HIGH SUGAR

Nutrition Facts	
Serving Size:	1 CUP
Amount Per Serving	
Calories:	110
Calories from Fat	9
Total Fat	1 gram
Saturated Fat	0
Cholesterol	0
Sodium	200 mg
Total Carbohydrate	25 grams
Dietary Fiber	1.2 gram
Soluble Fiber	
Insoluble Fiber	
Sugars	_12 grams (3 teaspoons)
Protein	2 grams

BARBARA'S SHREDDED WHEAT

Nutrition Facts

Serving Size: 2 Bisquits

Amount Per Serving
Calories: 140
Calories from Fat 10 calories
Total Fat 1 gram
Saturated Fat 0
Cholesterol 0 _
Sodium 0 mg
Potassium 160 mg
Total Carbohydrate 44 grams
Dietary Fiber 5 grams
Soluble fiber 1 gram
Insoluble fiber 4 grams
Sugars 0 grams__________
Other carbohydrate 31 grams
Protein 4 grams _________

POST
FROSTED SHREDDED WHEAT is VERY HIGH IN SUGAR!!!

Nutrition Facts

Serving Size: 1 CUP

Amount Per Serving cereal

Calories: 190

Calories from Fat 10

Total Fat 1 gram

Saturated Fat 0

Cholesterol 0

Sodium 10 mg

Potassium 170 mg

Total Carbohydrate 44 grams

Dietary Fiber 4 grams

Sugars 12 grams

Other carbohydrate 27 grams

Protein 4 grams

RICE KRISPIES is VERY HIGH IN AIR!	
Nutrition Facts	
Serving Size: 1 _ cups	
Servings Per Container: 12	
Amount Per Serving	
Calories: 120	160 calories
Calories from Fat 0	0 calories
Total Fat 0 grams	
Saturated Fat 0	
Cholesterol 0 _	
Sodium 350 mg	
Total Carbohydrate 29 grams	
Dietary Fiber 0 grams	
Sugars _3 grams_____	
Other carbohydrate 25 grams	
Protein 2 grams	

Although Rice Krispies have been around for years and has sustained its popularity, even in candy bars such as Nestle's Crunch, as a cereal it falls short nutritionally because it has zero fiber, not to mention its high sodium content. Select a cereal that has at least 3 grams or more of fiber, and resist getting junky foods that have toys in the box. TV is full of these seductive advertisements and your child has been primed to reach for candies that masquerade as food.

UNCLE SAM ORIGINAL

Nutrition Facts

Serving Size: _3/4 CUP

Amount Per Serving

Calories: 190	
Calories from Fat 40	
Total Fat 5 gram	
Saturated Fat 0.5 grams	
Cholesterol 0 _	
Sodium 135 mg	
Total Carbohydrate 38 grams	
Dietary Fiber 10 grams	
Soluble Fiber 2 grams	
Insoluble Fiber 8 grams	
Sugars less than 1 gram_____	
Protein 7 grams____________	

POST
100% BRAN

Nutrition Facts
Serving Size: 1/3 CUP
Amount Per Serving
Calories: 80
Calories from Fat 5
Total Fat 0.5 grams
Saturated Fat 0
Cholesterol 0 mg
Sodium 120
Potassium 270 mg
Total Carbohydrate 23 grams
Dietary Fiber 8 grams
Soluble Fiber 1 gram
Insoluble Fiber 7 grams
Sugars 7 grams
Other carbohydrate 8 grams
Protein 4 grams

Nutrition Facts
Serving Size 1 cup
Calories 140
Calories from Fat 10
Total Fat 1 gram
Saturated Fat 0 grams
Polyunsaturated 0.5 grams
Cholesterol 0 mg
Sodium 85 mg
Potassium 480 mg
Total Carbohydrate 24 grams
Dietary Fiber 10 grams
Soluble Fiber 1 gram
Insoluble Fiber 9 grams
Sugars 6 grams_
Protein 13 grams

WHEATIES

made with 100% Whole Wheat

Nutrition Facts

Serving Size: 1 cup

Servings Per Container: 17

Amount Per Serving
Calories: 110
Calories from Fat 10
Total Fat 1 gram
Saturated Fat 0.1 gram
Cholesterol 0
Sodium 190
Potassium 95
Total Carbohydrate 22 grams
Dietary Fiber 3 grams
Soluble Fiber
Insoluble Fiber
Sugars _4 grams___________
Other carbohydrate 17 grams
Protein 3 grams ___________

KASHI GO LEAN

Nutrition Facts

Serving Size: _ CUP

Amount Per Serving with _ cup skim milk

Calories: 110 150 calories

Calories from Fat 10 10 calories

Total Fat 1 gram

Saturated Fat 0 mg

Cholesterol 0 mg _

Sodium 200 _

Total Carbohydrate 24 grams

Dietary Fiber 3 grams

Sugars 5 grams __________

Protein 3 grams____________

Vitamin A 15% **Vitamin C** 25% **Vitamin D** 25%
Vitamin E 100% **Thiamin** 100 % **Riboflavin** 100%
Niacin 100 % **Iron** 100% **Calcium** 40%
Vitamin B6 100% **Vitamin** B12 110 %
Folic Acid 100% **Pantothenic Acid** 100%
Magnesium 10% **Zinc** 100% **Copper** 4%

KASHI
HEART TO HEART
(warm cinnamon oat cereal)

Nutrition Facts
Serving Size: 3/4 cup

Amount Per Serving

Calories: 120

Calories from Fat 15

Total Fat 1.5 grams

Saturated Fat 0

Cholesterol 0 _

Sodium 80 mg

Total Carbohydrate 25 grams

Dietary Fiber 5 grams

Soluble Fiber 1 gram

Insoluble Fiber 4 grams

Sugars 5 grams_________

Other carbohydrate 20 grams

Protein 4 grams__________

Thiamin % **Riboflavin** %
Niacin % **Iron** % **Calcium** %

FROOT LOOPS

Nutrition Facts

Serving Size: 1 CUP

Servings Per Container: 18

Amount Per Serving
Calories: 120
Calories from Fat 10
Total Fat 1 gram
Saturated Fat 0.5 grams
Cholesterol 0 _
Sodium 150 mg
Potassium 35 mg
Total Carbohydrate 28 grams
Dietary Fiber 1 gram
Sugars 15 grams_(almost 4 teaspoons)______
Other carbohydrate 12 grams
Protein 2 grams ____________

COCOA PUFFS
FROSTED CORN PUFFS

Nutrition Facts-This cereal along with FROOT LOOPS, LUCKY CHARMS, RICE CHEX AND CAP'N CRUNCH ARE SUGAR TOXIC AND NEED TO BE REMOVED FROM YOUR HOME

Serving Size: 1 CUP

Calories: 120

Calories from Fat 10

Total Fat 1 gram

Saturated Fat 0

Cholesterol 0 mg _

Sodium 190 mg

Total Carbohydrate 27 grams

Dietary Fiber 0 grams

Sugars _14 grams___________

Other carbohydrate 13 grams

Protein _1 gram____________

Thiamin % **Riboflavin** % **Niacin** % **Iron** % **Calcium** %

un-LUCKY CHARMS
Nutrition Facts
Serving Size 1 cup
Amount Per Serving About
Calories 120
Calories from Fat 10
Total Fat 1 gram
Saturated Fat 0
Polyunsaturated Fat 0
Monounsaturated Fat 0
Cholesterol 0
Sodium 210 mg
Total Carbohydrate 25 grams
Dietary Fiber 1 gram
Sugars 13 grams (over 3 teaspoons)
Other carbohydrate 11 grams
Protein 2 grams

Ingredients: Whole oat flour (includes oat bran), marshmallows (sugar, modified corn starch, corn syrup, Dextrose, gelatin, artificial flavors, yellow #5 & #6, red #40, blue #1) sugar, corn syrup, wheat starch, salt, color added, trisodium phosphate, calcium carbonate, zinc & iron, Vitamin C, niacin, B6, B2, B1, Vitamin A, folic acid, B12, Vitamin D, Vitamin E added to preserve freshness.

CAVEAT EMPTOR.....BUYER BEWARE!

RICE CHEX

Nutrition Facts
Serving Size 1 cup

Amount Per Serving About
Calories 120
Calories from Fat 0
Total Fat 0
Saturated Fat 0
Polyunsaturated Fat 0
Monounsaturated Fat 0
Cholesterol 0
Sodium 230 mg
Total Carbohydrate 27 grams
Dietary Fiber 0 !!!!
Sugars 2 grams
Other carbohydrates 25 grams
Protein 2 grams

CAP'N CRUNCH

Nutrition Facts
Serving Size _ cup
Amount Per Serving About
Calories 110
Calories from Fat 0
Total Fat 1.5 grams
Saturated Fat 0.5 grams
Cholesterol 0 mg
Sodium 210 mg
Potassium 35 mg
Total Carbohydrate 23 grams
Dietary Fiber 1 gram
Sugars 12 grams (3 teaspoons)
Other Carbohydrate 11 grams
Protein 1 gram

HERE ARE A FEW EXAMPLES OF OTHER BREAKFAST FOOD CHOICES

HOT CEREAL
CREAM OF WHEAT
(1/2 minute stovetop cooking)

Nutrition Facts

Serving Size 3 Tbs. make 1 cup

Amount Per Serving About

Calories 120

Calories from Fat 0

Total Fat 0 grams

Saturated Fat 0 gram

Cholesterol 0 mg

Sodium 0 mg

Total Carbohydrate 25 grams

Dietary Fiber 1 gram LOOK FOR A CEREAL WITH MORE FIBER!

Sugars 0 grams

Protein 3 grams

HERE IS A MORE WHOLESOME HOT CEREAL
STONE-BUHR 4 Grain[136]
(microwavable)

Nutrition Facts
Serving Size 1/3 cup
Servings Per Container 12
Amount Per Serving About
Calories 140
Calories from Fat 15
Total Fat 1.5 grams
Saturated Fat 0 gram _
Cholesterol 0 mg
Sodium 0 mg
Total Carbohydrate 31 grams
Dietary Fiber 5 grams
Sugars 0 grams
Protein 6 grams

Pancake mixes are very appealing because they appear to be easy to prepare. The problem with most mixes is they often contain ingredients you may wish to avoid. For example, pancake mixes almost all have excessive sodium and partially hydrogenated oils. Try the health-food stores for mixes high in whole grains or better yet, make your own pancakes from scratch. It's really easy. See page – for my recipe for buckwheat pancakes.

139 Stone Ground Mills, Inc. Seattle, WA 98126 (206)938-3478.

EGGS

Nutrition Facts
Serving Size: 1
Servings Per Container:

Amount Per Serving

Calories: 70

Calories from Fat 40

Total Fat 4.5 grams

Saturated Fat 1.5 grams

Cholesterol 210 mg

Sodium 65 mg

Total Carbohydrate 1 gram

Dietary Fiber 0

Sugars _0_________

Protein _6 grams____________

EGG BEATERS[137]

Nutrition Facts
Serving Size _ cup
Amount Per Serving About
Calories 30
Calories from Fat 0
Total Fat 0 grams
Saturated Fat 0 _
Cholesterol 0 mg
Sodium 110 mg
Total Carbohydrate 1 gram
Dietary Fiber 0 grams
Sugars less than 1 gram
Protein 5 grams

140 The egg substitute ***Ener G Egg Replacer,*** found in many natural food market, is for people who cannot use regular eggs in their diets and who want a replacer that's animal protein-free. It can be used to replace both whole eggs and eggs whites in bakery goods, mayonnaise, and meringues. It is not designed to be used by itself in scrambled eggs or omelets. It contains potato starch, tapioca flour, leavening and carbohydrate gum. This mixture is particularly good in baked products such as muffins, cookies, and fruit breads.

SNACKS

If you learn to read labels you can find many delicious snack crackers that have high nutritional value that children enjoy. Here are a few examples, but limit crackers to only a few, since the combination of grapes, juice, raisins, and crackers often leads to a poor appetite.

Reduced fat Triscuit Wafers have 3 grams of fat compared with 5 grams in Original Triscuit Wafers. For a product to be called reduced, it must contain 40% less fat than regular Triscuit crackers. Check the sodium content (180 mg). Check the calories per serving (130 mg). This is a good sodium to calorie balance. Fiber content is a respectable 4 mg, however, the label does not tell us how much of the fiber is soluble or insoluble.

TRISCUIT

Baked Whole Wheat Wafers
Reduced Fat 40% Less Fat Than Original Triscuit

Nutrition Facts
Serving Size: 8 wafers
Servings Per Container: 8

Amount Per Serving
Calories: 130
Calories from Fat 25
Total Fat 3 grams
Saturated Fat 0.5 grams
Cholesterol 0
Sodium 180 mg
Total Carbohydrate 24 grams
Dietary Fiber 4 grams
Sugars 0
Protein 3 grams
Vitamin C 0% **Vitamin A** 0% **Iron** 10 % **Calcium** 0 %

RY KRISP

Nutrition Facts
Serving Size: 2 CRACKERS
Servings Per Container: 17

Amount Per Serving
Calories: 60
Calories from Fat 10
% **Daily Value**
Total Fat 1.5 GRAMS
Saturated Fat 0 GRAMS
Cholesterol 0 MG
Sodium 90 MG
Total Carbohydrate 10 GRAMS
Dietary Fiber 3 GRAMS
Sugars 0 GRAMS_______
Protein 1 GRAM ___________

A nutritious cracker is an excellent after school snack. Serve them along with non-fat string cheese, cherry tomatoes, sliced cucumbers, raw carrots or celery and a favorite fruit, such as apple, banana or orange slices.

CRUNCHMASTER MULTI-GRAIN CRACKERS GLUTEN FREE

Serving Size-7 Crackers

Calories-60

Calories from fat-15

Total Fat-1.5 grams

Saturated Fat-0

Trans Fat-0

Cholesterol-0

Sodium-65 mg

Potassium-40 grams

Total Carbohydrate-11 grams

Dietary Fiber- 1 gram

Sugars-1 gram

Protein- 1 gram

NOW COMPARE REDUCED FAT TRISCUITS AND RY KRISP WITH OTHER CRACKERS:

MANISCHEWITZ

MATZO - CRACKER MINIATURES

Nutrition Facts
Serving Size 13
Servings Per Container 8
Amount Per Serving About
Calories 110
Calories from Fat 0
Total Fat 0.5 grams
Saturated Fat 0 _ _
Cholesterol 0
Sodium 0
Total Carbohydrate 25 grams
Dietary Fiber 1 gram
Sugars 1 gram
Protein 3 grams

These crackers are better than Goldfish crackers. Check the Nutritional Facts label the next time you shop. Goldfish contains 6 grams of fat, 230 mg sodium, and no fiber! DON'T FEED THESE CRACKERS TO YOUR CHILDREN or use them as "shut-up" tools!!

These crackers should also be on the "no-no" list.

CHEEZ-IT

(White Cheddar)

Nutrition Facts

Serving Size: 26 crackers

Amount Per Serving

Calories: 150

Calories from Fat 70

Total Fat 7 grams

Saturated Fat 1.5 grams

Cholesterol < 1 mg _

Sodium 280 mg _

Total Carbohydrate 18 grams

Dietary Fiber < 1 gram

Sugars < 1 gram_______

Protein 3 grams ________

QUAKER salt free RICE CAKES

Nutrition Facts
Serving Size 1
Servings Per Container 14
Amount Per Serving About
Calories 35
Calories from Fat 0
Total Fat 0 grams
Saturated Fat 0 _
Cholesterol 0 mg
Sodium 0 mg
Total Carbohydrate 7 grams
Dietary Fiber 0 grams
Sugars 0 grams
Protein 1 gram

Ingredients: Whole grain brown rice

To add more fiber, use a high fiber spread, such as hummus.

Snyder's of
HANOVER SOURDOUGH
UNSALTED HARD PRETZELS

Nutrition Facts
Serving Size 1
Servings Per Container 15

Amount Per Serving About
Calories 100
Calories from Fat 0
Total Fat 0 grams
Saturated Fat 0 grams _
Cholesterol 0 mg
Sodium 90 mg
Total Carbohydrate 22 grams
Dietary Fiber 1 gram
Sugars 0 grams
Protein 3 grams

PADERINOS reduced fat TORTILLA CHIPS "Original"
40% less fat than regular tortilla chips

Nutrition Facts
Serving Size 1 oz (14 chips)
Servings Per Container

Amount Per Serving About
Calories 130
Calories from Fat 40
Total Fat 4 grams
Saturated Fat 0.5 grams
Cholesterol 0 mg
Sodium 125 mg
Total Carbohydrate 20 grams
Dietary Fiber 1 gram
Sugars 0
Protein 2 grams

Ingredients: Corn, Rice, Corn & Canola oil, Salt.
Granny Goose Foods, Inc. Oakland, CA 94603

ORVILLE REDENBACHER'S POPPING CORN
ORIGINAL
100% whole grain

NUTRITION FACTS
Serving Size: 3 Tbs. (unpopped)—makes about 6 cups popped

Calories: 120	
	Calories from Fat: 10
Total Fat: 1.5 grams	
	Saturated Fat: 0
	Trans Fats: 0
	Polyunsaturated Fat: 0.5 grams
	Monounsaturated Fat 0
Cholesterol: 0	
Sodium: 0	
Total Carbohydrate: 29 grams	
	Dietary fiber 5 grams
Protein: 4 grams	

Prepare in Hot Air Popper

1. **Pour level ½ cup popcorn into popping chamber.**
2. **Set cover into groove on popping chamber.**
3. **Place cup used to measure popcorn into opening on top of cover**

4. **Set 4-quart or larger heat-proof bowl under popping chute to collect popped corn.**
5. **Plug unit into 120 volt AC electrical outlet. Popping will be completed within 2-3 minutes after popping begins.**
6. **Reseal jar to retain moisture and freshness and store at room temperature.**

NOW DON'T RUIN IT BY POURING MELTED BUTTER AND SALT OVER THIS NUTRITIOUS AND FUN SNACK!

COMPARE WITH "MOVIE POP CORN"

NUTRITION FACTS
Calories in Movie Theater Popcorn -Large
Serving size: 1 serving
Amount per Serving
Calories: 664
Total Fat: 31 grams
Saturated Fat: 27 grams
Polyunsaturated Fat: 0
Monounsaturated Fat: 0
Cholesterol: 0
Sodium: 443 mg
Potassium: 0
Total Carbohydrate: 75 grams
Dietary Fiber: 9 grams
Sugars: 0
Protein: 13 grams

Now wash this down with a Large Soda: 65 grams of sugar (over 16 teaspoons of sugar).

BREADS

OROWEAT LIGHT BREAD

All breads are high in sodium. Look for breads with a high fiber content. For example, Orowheat Light Bread has a fiber content of 5 grams per serving and no fat. Most breads contain on 1-2 grams of fiber per portion

WONDER BREAD

Nutrition Facts-WHAT HAPPENED TO THE FIBER?
Serving Size 1 Slice
Servings Per Container 24

Amount Per Serving About	
Calories	70
Calories from Fat	0
Total Fat	1 gram
Saturated Fat	0 grams
Polyunsaturated Fat	0 grams
Monounsaturated Fat	0 grams
Cholesterol	0 mg
Sodium	150 mg
Total Carbohydrate	14 grams
Dietary Fiber	0 grams
Sugars	1 gram
Protein	2 grams

Children love white bread, white rice and white pasta, but whole grain foods are more nutritious and take longer to turn into sugar. Try to introduce whole grain foods. Milling rains removes the fiber-rich outer layer along with B vitamins and phytochemicals-those non-nutritive substances that have subtle effects on health.

WHOLE WHEAT BREAD
Nutrition Facts
Serving Size: 1 slice
Calories: 60
Calories from Fat 10
Total Fat 1 gram
Saturated Fat 0 grams
Cholesterol 0 mg
Sodium 120 mg
Total Carbohydrate 11 grams
Dietary Fiber 2 grams
Sugars 1 gram
Protein 3 grams

SEARCH FOR A BREAD WITH AT LEAST 3 grams OF FIBER.

WHOLE WHEAT PITA BREAD
(Pocket Bread)

Nutrition Facts
Serving Size 1 pita
Amount Per Serving About
Calories 130
Calories from Fat 10
Total Fat 1 gram
Saturated Fat 0 grams
Polyunsaturated Fat 0.5 grams
Cholesterol 0 mg
Sodium 340 mg
Total Carbohydrate 27 grams
Dietary Fiber 4.7 grams
Sugars 0.5 grams
Protein 6 grams

La Tortilla Factory[140] organic KING SIZE Corn Tortillas

Nutrition Facts
Serving Size 2
Amount Per Serving About
Calories 120
Calories from Fat 9
Total Fat 1 gram
Saturated Fat <0.5 gram
Cholesterol 0 mg
Sodium 0 mg
Total Carbohydrate 25 grams
Dietary Fiber 2 grams
Sugars <0.5 grams
Protein 2 grams

Try a tortilla wrap: Place a tortilla between two dampened paper towels. Microwave on high until warm. Sprinkle low or reduced fat mozzarella cheese (about 1 tablespoon) over the center of the warmed tortilla. Spoon salsa over the cheese. Fold the tortilla as a "blinza" or crepe. Microwave for another 20 seconds. Enjoy this nutritious snack, but don't burn your mouth!

[141] La Tortilla Factory 3654 Standish Ave. Santa Rosa, CA 95407 800-446-1516.

ORGANIC
TRICOLOR QUINOA
(Gluten Free)

NUTRITION FACTS
Serving Size ¼ cup

Calories: 160	
	Calories from Fat: 25
Total Fat: 2.5 grams	
	Saturated Fat: 0
	Trans Fat: 0
Cholesterol: 0	
Sodium: 0	
Total Carbohydrate: 30 grams	
Total Fiber: 3 grams	
	Sugars: 3 grams
Protein: 6 grams	

HODSON MILL
COUSCOUS
(Whole Wheat)

NUTRITION FACTS
Serving size: 1/3 cup

Amount Per Serving	
Calories: 210	
Calories from Fat: 10	
Total Fat: 1 gram	
Saturated Fat: 0	
Cholesterol: 0	
Sodium: 0	
Total Carbohydrate: 47 grams	
Dietary Fiber: 5 grams	
Sugars: 1 gram	
Protein: 8 grams	

BUTTER AND OTHER SPREADS

COMPARE BUTTER WITH THE FOLLOWING SPREADS

BUTTER

Nutrition Facts
Serving Size 1 Tbs.
Servings Per Container 32

Amount Per Serving About
Calories 100
Calories from Fat 100
Total Fat 11 grams
Saturated Fat 7 grams !!!!!!
Cholesterol 30 mg
Sodium 90 mg
Total Carbohydrate 0 grams
Dietary Fiber 0 grams
Sugars 0 grams
Protein 0 grams

EXTRA VIRGIN OLIVE OIL
(Although not a "spread" it's included here so you can compare it with butter)

Nutrition Facts
Serving Size 1 Tbs.

Amount Per Serving About
Calories 120
Calories from Fat 120
Total Fat 14 grams
Saturated Fat 2 gram
Polyunsaturated Fat 1 gram
Monounsaturated Fat 10 grams
Cholesterol 0 mg
Sodium 0 mg
Total Carbohydrate 0 grams
Dietary Fiber 0 gram
Sugars 0 grams
Protein 0 grams

PROMISE ULTRA SPREAD

Vegetable Oil Spread

70% Less Fat **than margarine**

Nutrition Facts

Serving Size 1 Tbs

Amount Per Serving About	
Calories 30	
	Calories from Fat 30
Total Fat 3.5 grams	
	Saturated Fat 0 grams
	Polyunsaturated Fat 1 gram
	Monounsaturated Fat 2 grams
Cholesterol 0 mg	
Sodium 60 mg	
Total Carbohydrate 0 grams	
	Dietary Fiber 0 grams
	Sugars 0 grams
Protein 0 grams	

Benicol *Light* Spread

Nutrition Facts
Serving Size 1 container (8 grams)
Servings Per Container 21
Amount Per Serving About
Calories 30
Calories from Fat 30
Total Fat 3 grams
Saturated Fat 0 grams
Polyunsaturated Fat 1.5 grams
Monounsaturated Fat 1.0 grams
Cholesterol 0 mg
Sodium 65 mg
Total Carbohydrate 0 grams
Dietary Fiber 0 grams
Sugars 0 grams
Protein 0 grams
Vitamin A 10% **Vitamin D** 10% **Calcium** 0% **Vitamin E** 4%

I CAN'T BELIEVE IT'S NOT BUTTER 60% VEGETABLE FAT SPREAD

Nutrition Facts

Serving Size 1 tbs.

Amount Per Serving About
Calories 80
Calories from Fat 80
Total Fat 9 grams
Saturated Fat 1.5 grams *
Polyunsaturated Fat 2 grams
Monounsaturated Fat 2 grams
Cholesterol 0 mg
Sodium 100 mg
Total Carbohydrate 0 grams
Dietary Fiber 0 grams
Sugars 0 grams
Protein 0 grams

KRAFT MAYO REAL MAYONNAISE

Nutrition Facts

Serving Size 1 Tbs.

Servings Per Container

Amount Per Serving About
Calories 100
Calories from Fat 100
Total Fat 11 grams
Saturated Fat 2 grams
Cholesterol 5 mg
Sodium 75 mg
Total Carbohydrate 0 grams
Dietary Fiber 0 grams
Sugars 0 grams
Protein 0 grams

Compare the other spreads with Kraft Real Mayonnaise. Note especially the calories from fat.

KRAFT *LIGHT* MAYO

Nutrition Facts
Serving Size 1 Tbs.
Calories 50
Calories from Fat 45
Total Fat 5 grams
Saturated Fat 1 gram
Cholesterol 5 mg
Sodium 90 mg
Total Carbohydrate 2 grams
Dietary Fiber 0 grams
Sugars less than 1 gram
Protein 0 grams

This is a relatively better-tasting low fat spread.

COMPARE THE AMOUNT OF SATURATED FATS BETWEEN REGULAR CREAM CHEESE, LITE, AND NON-FAT CREAM CHEESE.

DAIRY AND DAIRY SUBSTITUTES

CREAM CHEESE

Nutrition Facts
Serving Size 1 oz 30
Servings Per Container

Amount Per Serving

Calories 100

Calories from Fat 90

Total Fat grams 10 grams

Saturated Fat grams 6 grams

Cholesterol mg 30 mg

Sodium 95 mg

Total Carbohydrate grams <1 gram

Dietary Fiber 0 grams

Sugars grams 0 grams

Protein grams 2 grams

Vitamin A 15% **Vitamin C** 0%
Calcium 2%

LITE CREAM CHEESE

Nutrition Facts

Serving Size 1 oz (30 grams)

Amount Per Serving About
Calories 60
Calories from Fat 40
Total Fat 5 grams
Saturated Fat 3 grams
Cholesterol 10 mg
Sodium 160 mg
Total Carbohydrate 2 grams
Dietary Fiber 0 grams
Sugars 1 gram
Protein 3 grams

FAT-FREE CREAM CHEESE

Nutrition Facts
Serving Size 1 oz.
Amount Per Serving About
Calories 30
Calories from Fat 0
Total Fat 0 grams
Saturated Fat 0 grams
Cholesterol 0 mg
Sodium 150 mg
Total Carbohydrate 1 gram
Dietary Fiber 0 grams
Sugars 1 gram
Protein 5 grams
Vitamin A 8% **Calcium** 8%

WHOLE VITAMIN D MILK

2% MILK

(Reduced Fat)

2% IS NOT LOW FAT!

Nutrition Facts

Serving Size 1 cup (236ml.)

Amount Per Serving
Calories 160
Calories from Fat 70
Total Fat grams 8 grams
Saturated Fat 5 grams
Cholesterol 35 mg
Sodium mg 125 mg
Total Carbohydrate 13 grams
Dietary Fiber 0 grams
Sugars grams 12 grams
Protein grams 8 grams
Vitamin A 10% **Vitamin C** 2% **Vitamin D** 25% **Calcium** 30% **Iron** 0%

1% MILK
(Low Fat)

Nutrition Facts
Serving Size 8 flu oz.
Amount Per Serving
Calories 130
Calories from Fat 45
Total Fat 5 grams
Saturated Fat 3 grams
Cholesterol 25mg
Sodium 130mg
Total Carbohydrate 13 grams
Dietary Fiber 0 grams
Sugars 13 grams_
Protein 10 grams
Vitamin A 10% **Vitamin C** 4%
Vitamin D 25% **Calcium** 40%
Iron 0%

These are the Nutritional Facts from a carton of Grade A pasteurized, homogenized 1% low fat milk.

As you can see, milk is an excellent source of protein and calcium. There is no iron in milk or yogurt and that is why a diet too high in dairy contributes to anemia and because there is no fiber in milk, constipation is common in children who consume too much milk at the expense of vegetables and fruit. Note the sodium content of milk and other dairy products, and you will readily see why added salt is unnecessary to the diet. Two glasses of milk and two slices of white or whole wheat bread already contributes 670 milligrams of sodium to a child's diet.

FAT FREE MILK
(SKIM)

Nutrition Facts

Serving Size 8 fl oz.

Servings Per Container 4

Amount Per Serving

Calories 130

Calories from Fat 20

Total Fat 2.5g

Saturated Fat 1.5g

Cholesterol 15 mg

Sodium 160 mg

Total Carbohydrate 16 grams

Dietary Fiber 0 grams

Sugars 15grams________

Protein 11grams

Vitamin A 10% **Vitamin C** 4%
Vitamin D 25% **Calcium** 40%
Iron 0%

VANILLA RICE DREAM

Nutrition Facts	
Serving Size 8 fl oz.	
Servings Per Container 4	
Amount Per Serving	
Calories 130	
Calories from Fat 20	
Total Fat 2 grams	
Saturated Fat 0 grams	
Cholesterol 0 mg	
Sodium 90 mg	
Total Carbohydrate 28 grams	
Dietary Fiber 0 grams	
Sugars 12 grams_	
Protein 1 gram	
Vitamin A 0%	**Vitamin C** 0%
Vitamin D 0%	**Calcium** 2%
Iron 0%	**Vitamin E** 4%

Ingredients: Filtered water, Brown rice, (Partially milled) Expeller Pressed Oleic, Safflower oil, Vanilla, Sea salt

Rice dream has become a popular substitute for milk. Look carefully at the Nutritional Food Label and note that the protein content is only 1 gram per serving. This is in contrast with the 9 grams found in fat free milk! Children need protein and if Rice Dream is used as a substitute for milk, it is extremely important for the baby or child to get adequate protein from another source. The same is true for Vitamin D and calcium. Milk is a rich source of both, while Rice Dream is deficient in both nutrients. If for some reason you are inclined to give Rice Dream to your child, be certain to use the enriched form (with Vitamin A, D & Calcium.) Older children and young adults also need these nutrients. Children 10 to 21 years of age get most of their calcium during those years. These are the years when sufficient calcium storage along with Vitamin D, a reduced sodium diet and exercise can prevent or delay the onset of osteoporosis.

Nutrition Facts
Serving Size 8 fl oz.
Servings Per Container 4

Amount Per Serving	
Calories 90	
	Calories from Fat 0
Total Fat 0 grams	
	Saturated Fat 0 grams
Cholesterol less than 5 mg	
Sodium 120 mg	
Total Carbohydrate 12 grams	
	Dietary Fiber 0 grams
	Sugars 12 grams_
Protein 9 grams	

Vitamin A 10% **Vitamin C** 4%
Vitamin D 25% **Calcium** 40%
Iron 0%

BEVERAGES

GATORADE

This "sport drink" has enjoyed popularity as a "re-hydration" fluid. Many doctors recommend it for children who are vomiting or have diarrhea, in order to prevent dehydration. Gatorade may be good for the long distance runner, but it's not advisable to give this drink to either healthy or ill children. It's too high in sodium for the healthy child and its high sugar content may increase diarrhea.

GATORADE

Nutrition Facts
Serving Size 8 fl oz.
Servings Per Container
Amount Per Serving
Calories 50
Calories from Fat 0
Total Fat 0 grams
Saturated Fat 0grams
Cholesterol 0 mg
Sodium 110 mg
Potassium 30 mg
Total Carbohydrate 14 grams
Dietary Fiber 0 grams
Sugars 14 grams_
Protein 0 grams

V8 JUICE
Nutrition Facts
Serving Size 1 Can (340 ml)
Servings Per Container 1
Amount Per Serving
Calories 70
Calories from Fat 0
Total Fat 0 grams
Saturated Fat 0 grams
Cholesterol 0 mg
Sodium 880 mg
Potassium 780 mg
Total Carbohydrate 15 grams
Dietary Fiber 2 grams
Sugars 11 grams
Protein 2 grams

V8 JUICE

WOW, I could of had a cup of salt water! CAMPBELL'S TOMATO JUICE

This high sodium beverage should not be given to children. There are many other wholesome choices. Don't forget water. It's an excellent beverage.

CAPRI-SUN
"ALL NATURAL"
FRUIT PUNCH JUICE DRINK

Nutrition Facts	
Serving Size 1 Can (340 ml)	
Servings Per Container 1	
Amount Per Serving	
Calories 70	
Calories from Fat 0	
Total Fat 0 grams	
Saturated Fat 0 grams	
Cholesterol 0 mg	
Sodium 1230 mg	
Total Carbohydrate 13grams	
Dietary Fiber 2 grams	
Sugars 9 grams_	
Protein 2 grams	

WHAT IS IN THIS POPULAR DRINK?

Ingredients: Water, high fructose corn syrup, pineapple, water extracted orange, grapefruit and peach juice concentrate, citric acid, natural flavor.

In other words-pure sugar water! Avoid punch, and fruit "drinks." Kool Aid, Kool Aid Bursts, Hi-C, or soft drink mixes. These products are packaged and advertised heavily on TV to attract children. Protect your children from these beverages and send your child to school with a more nourishing beverage.

"Twice the Fruit" Fat-Free Yogurt
(Safeway Brand)

Nutrition Facts
Serving Size 1 POUCH
Servings Per Container 1

Amount Per Serving
Calories 100
Calories from Fat 0
Total Fat 0 grams
Saturated Fat 0 grams
Cholesterol 0 mg
Sodium 20 mg
Total Carbohydrate 26 grams
Dietary Fiber 0 grams
Sugars 26 grams_ (over 6 teaspoons sugar)
Protein 0 grams
Vitamin A 10% **Vitamin C** 4%
Vitamin D 25% **Calcium** 40% **Iron** 0%

"Twice the Fruit" Fat-Free Yogurt
Nutrition Facts
Serving Size 1 (227g)
Servings Per Container about 1
Amount Per Serving
Calories 260
Total Fat 0g
Saturated Fat 0g
Cholesterol 5mg
Sodium 160mg
Total Carbohydrate 55 grams
Dietary Fiber 0 grams
Sugars 52 grams
Protein 11grams
Vitamin A Vitamin C 2%
Calcium 40% **Iron** 0%

———Note that the nutritional value of milk is about the same as yogurt except for the added sugar which accounts for the extra calories. Plain non-fat yogurt has the same amount of calories as non-fat milk. Milk has 15 grams of milk-sugar (lactose) versus 55 grams in this yogurt which means that an extra 40 grams of sugar[142]has been added. Try instead to add some fresh fruit or berries to plain yogurt. This will give you fewer refined sugar calories, more vitamins, and some fiber. Calcium is reported in percent, but we usually think in terms of milligrams of calcium. This is confusing to most shoppers who are trying to provide sufficient calcium. In this case, 40% is equal to 320mg of elemental calcium.

[142] One teaspoon of granulated sugar is about 4 grams and contains 15 calories

BEN & JERRY'S LOW FAT FROZEN YOGURT

Nutrition Facts
Serving Size 1/2 cup (89g)
Servings Per Container 4
Amount Per Serving
Calories 150
Calories from Fat 0
Total Fat 0 grams______
Saturated Fat 0 grams
Cholesterol 5mg
Sodium 80mg
Total Carbohydrate 32 grams
Dietary Fiber 0 grams
Sugars 24 grams
Protein 3 grams
Vitamin A 2% **Vitamin C** 0%
Calcium 10% **Iron** 2%

Low Fat Frozen Yogurt contains about 3 grams of fat, of which two are from saturated fat. Regular Ben & Jerry's Ice Cream contains a whopping 28 grams of fat per serving.

This Nutrition Facts label is included to illustrate how easy it is to find delicious low fat substitutes for traditionally high fat foods or desserts.

Remember that LOW FAT doesn't mean LOW CALORIE nor does it mean "healthy." It should not mean, "Now I can eat, ' The whole thing.' " Keep your sugary dessert portions small, and never use, "non-fat" as permission to "pig out." Non-fat often means high sugar calories. And calories do count!

For those of you who are regular yogurt lovers, remember: Fruit-flavored yogurt is made with jam, a poor source of nutrients. The jam adds the equivalent of 8-9 teaspoons of sugar per cup! Instead, add fresh fruit to plain yogurt.

REGULAR SOUR CREAM

Loaded with artery-clogging saturated fat.

Nutrition Facts

Serving Size 2 tbs.

Calories 60	
	Calories from Fat 50
Total Fat 6 grams	
	Saturated Fat 4 grams
Cholesterol 25 mg	
Sodium 15 mg	
Total Carbohydrate 1 gram	
	Dietary Fiber 0 grams
	Sugars 1 gram
Protein 1 gram	

Vitamin A 4% **Vitamin C** 0%
Calcium 2% **Iron** 0%

NATURALLY YOURS[142] *FAT FREE* SOUR CREAM

Nutrition Facts
Serving Size 2 Tbs.
Servings Per Container 15
Amount Per Serving About
Calories 20
Calories from Fat 0
Total Fat 0 grams
Cholesterol 0 mg
Sodium 50 mg
Total Carbohydrate 3 grams
Dietary Fiber 0 grams
Sugars 2 grams
Protein 1 gram
Vitamin 4%A **Vitamin C** 0%
Calcium 4% **Iron** 0%

Experiment with the taste of the many new fat free sour cream choices.

143 Distributed by in STAR Inc. 5956 Sherry Lane Dallas, TX 75225 Tel: 800-441-3321.

KNUDSEN *FREE* FAT FREE SOUR CREAM

Nutrition Facts

Serving Size 2 Tbs.

Amount Per Serving About

Calories 35

Calories from Fat 0

Total Fat 0 grams

Cholesterol less than 5 mg

Sodium 25 mg

Total Carbohydrate 6 grams

Dietary Fiber 0 grams

Sugars 2 grams

Protein 2 grams

Vitamin A 4% **Vitamin C** 0%
Calcium 4% **Iron** 0%

AMERICAN OR CHEDDAR CHEESE

Choose a cheese lower in saturated fat.

Nutrition Facts

Serving Size 1 oz. or 1 slice

Servings Per Container 12

Amount Per Serving About
Calories 120
Calories from Fat 90
Total Fat 10 grams
Saturated Fat 6 grams
Unsaturated 4 grams
Cholesterol 25 mg
Sodium 180 mg
Total Carbohydrate 1 gram
Dietary Fiber 0 grams
Sugars grams 0 grams
Protein grams 7 grams
Vitamin A 6% **Vitamin C** 0% **Calcium** 20% **Iron** 0%

***ALPINE LACE* REDUCED FAT SWISS CHEESE**

(25% Less Total Fat & 53% Less Sodium)

Nutrition Facts

Serving Size 1 oz.

Amount Per Serving About
Calories 110
Calories from Fat 60
Total Fat 7 Grams
Saturated Fat 4.5 grams
Cholesterol 25 mg
Sodium 140 mg
Total Carbohydrate 1 grams
Dietary Fiber 0 grams
Sugars 1 grams
Protein 8 grams
Vitamin A 6% **Vitamin C** 0%
Calcium 25% **Iron** 0%

HEALTHY CHOICE LOW FAT MOZZARELLA CHEESE
(STRING CHEESE)

Nutrition Facts
Serving Size 1 Piece
Servings Per Container 10

Amount Per Serving About

Calories 50

Calories from Fat

Total Fat 1.5 grams

Saturated Fat 1 gram

Cholesterol less than 5 mg

Sodium 220 mg

Total Carbohydrate 1 gram

Dietary Fiber 0 grams

Sugars 0 grams

Protein 8 grams

Vitamin A 4% **Vitamin C** 0%
Calcium 20% **Iron** 0%

Shredded non-fat or low-fat mozzarella cheese is excellent as a "melt" over a whole wheat English Muffin. To make pizza, put pizza sauce over the muffin, then cheese. Microwave until cheese melts.

LOW FAT (1%) COTTAGE CHEESE

Although a bit high in sodium, this is an excellent high protein after school snack along with fresh fruit or berries for extra vitamins and fiber. It may come as a surprise to you that there is little calcium in cottage cheese.

FRUIT

Nutrition Facts
Serving Size _ 1 cup

Amount Per Serving
Calories 72
Calories from Fat 9
Total Fat 1 gram
Saturated Fat <1 gram
Cholesterol 4 mg
Sodium 400mg
Total Carbohydrate 3 grams
Dietary Fiber 0 grams
Sugars 1 gram_
Protein 12 grams
Vitamin A 4% **Vitamin C** 0%
Calcium 2% **Iron** 0%

FROZEN BIG VALLEY CALIFORNIA MIXED FRUIT

PEACHES, CANTALOUPE AND HONEYDEW MELON, RED SEEDLESS GRAPES

If or when seasonal fruit is not available, this is an excellent second choice. It is more nutritious than canned fruit.

Nutrition Facts	
Serving Size _ 1 cup	
Servings Per Container 18	
Amount Per Serving	
Calories 60	
Calories from Fat 0	
Total Fat 0 grams	
Saturated Fat 0 grams	
Cholesterol 0 mg	
Sodium 0 mg	
Total Carbohydrate 14 grams	
Dietary Fiber 2 grams	
Sugars 8 grams_	
Protein 1 gram	
Vitamin A 20%	**Vitamin C** 150%

DRIED* BING CHERRIES

*Other dried fruit such as prune, apricot, pear, apple and peach are available at most supermarket and health food stores. Banana chips are deep fried and should be avoided. They are much closer to potato chips than bananas or dried fruit. One ounce of dried chips has nearly 10 grams of fat, mostly saturated, coming often from coconut oil. These chips are made from bananas that are picked green before the starch has had time to change to sugar. Sugar is added to make them taste sweet.

TRADER JOE'S* DRIED PITTED CALIFORNIA BING CHERRIES

Nutrition Facts
Serving Size 1/3 cup
Servings Per Container 6

Amount Per Serving
Calories 140
Calories from Fat 0
Total Fat 0 grams
Saturated Fat 0 grams
Cholesterol 0 mg
Sodium 0 mg
Total Carbohydrate 34 grams
Dietary Fiber 2 grams
Sugars 25 grams_ ???? How much of this is sugar added??
Protein 1 gram
Vitamin A 2% **Vitamin C** 0%

*Distributed and sold exclusively by Trader Joe's, So. Pasadena, CA91031

No preservatives. No artificial colors or flavors.

Great for snacks or to bake into muffins, breads and cookies (just as you would use raisins). They add flavor to home made trail mixes and fruit salads.

TRADER JOE'S DRIED BLUEBERRIES

Nutrition Facts	
Serving Size 1/4 cup	
Servings Per Container 5	
Amount Per Serving	
Calories 160	
Calories from Fat 0	
Total Fat 0 grams	
Saturated Fat 0 grams	
Cholesterol 0 mg	
Sodium 0 mg	
Total Carbohydrate 38 grams	
Dietary Fiber 5 grams	
Sugars 20 grams_ ?? How much Fructose is added??	
Protein <1 gram	
Vitamin A 0% **Vitamin C** 0%	
Calcium 2% **Iron** 2%	

Ingredients: Blueberries, Fructose, Malic Acid, Sunflower Oil.

Dried fruit is high in fiber and are good for snacks or to bake into muffins, breads and cookies (just as you would raisins). I found the dried bing cherries more flavorful than the dried blueberries. Add dried fruit to cereals to enhance flavor and add fiber.

There is no way to tell from this label how much fructose is added sugar.

COMPARE CANNED VEGETABLES FOR NUTRITIONAL VALUE

S&W PEELED TOMATOES READY CUT

Nutrition Facts	
Serving Size	1/2 cup
Amount Per Serving About	
Calories	25
Calories from Fat	0
Total Fat	0 grams
Saturated Fat	0 gram
Cholesterol	0 mg
Sodium	190 mg
Potassium	150mg
Total Carbohydrate	4 grams
Dietary Fiber	1 gram
Sugars	4 grams
Protein	1 gram
VITAMIN A 20% **VITAMIN C** 15%	
CALCIUM 4% **IRON** 15%	

Buy the no-salt added canned vegetables. When you have a choice, always try to select the brand with the least added sodium.

S&W PEELED TOMATOS
NO SALT ADDED
READY CUT

Nutrition Facts
Serving Size ½ cup
Servings Per Container 3

Calories 25
Calories from Fat 0
Total Fat 0 grams
Saturated Fat 0 grams
Cholesterol 0 mg
Sodium 30 mg
Potassium 105mg
Total Carbohydrate 4 grams
Dietary Fiber 1 grams
Sugars 3 grams
Protein 1 gram
VITAMIN A 20% **VITAMIN C** 15%
CALCIUM 0% **IRON** 10%

HEINZ
VEGETARIAN BEANS IN RICE & TOMATO SAUCE

Nutrition Facts
Serving Size ½ cup

Amount Per Serving About	
Calories 140	
	Calories from Fat 0
Total Fat 0 grams	
	Saturated Fat 0 gram _
Cholesterol 0 mg	
Sodium 480 mg (Look for something similar with less sodium)	
Total Carbohydrate 27 grams	
	Dietary Fiber 5 grams
	Sugars 14 grams---check labels to see whether there are any other brands with less sugar added.
Protein 6 grams	

GOOSE VALLEY-FAMILY BLEND

Brown & Wild Rice-Fusion

100% Whole Grain

Nutrition Facts
Serving Size: ¼ cup
Calories 150
Calories from Fat 10
Total Fat 1.5 grams
Saturated Fat 0
Trans Fat 0
Cholesterol 0
Sodium 0
Total Carbohydrate 35 grams
Dietary Fiber 4 grams
Sugars 2 grams
Protein 5 grams

RICE A RONI

(CHICKEN FLAVORED)[143]

Nutrition Facts

Serving Size 2.5 oz. or 1 cup prepared

Amount Per Serving About	
Calories 300 prepared	
Total Fat 9 grams	
	Calories from Fat 80 (prepared)
Sodium 1060 mg (prepared)	
	Saturated Fat grams
	Trans Fat 1.5 grams
Cholesterol 5 mg	
Dietary Fiber 1 gram	
Total Fat 1 grams*	
	Saturated Fat 1.5 grams
	Sodium 1090 mg. (prepared)
Total Carbohydrate 50 grams	
	Dietary Fiber 2 grams
	Sugars 3 grams
Protein 7 grams	
FOLATE 25% **CALCIUM** 2% **IRON** 10%	

144 DON'T LOOK FOR THE CHICKEN. THERE ISN'T ANY.

BUMBLE BEE
TUNA SALAD
(MIXED AND READY TO EAT)
FAT FREE

Nutrition Facts
Serving Size 1 can
Servings Per Container 1
Amount Per Serving About
Calories 70
Calories from Fat 0
Total Fat 0 grams
Saturated Fat 0 grams _
Cholesterol 15 mg
Sodium 380 mg
Total Carbohydrate 10 grams
Dietary Fiber 0 grams
Sugars 5 grams
Protein 7 grams

Limit tuna to once a week because of the small mercury present.

Try the Bumble Bee Chunk Light Tuna in Water (easy to open cans). They only have 1 gram of fat and 15 grams of protein. Sodium is a bit high. They make a good school lunch along with low sodium crackers, celery, cherry tomatoes and a piece of fresh fruit.

DENNISON'S *REDUCED FAT* CHILI CON CARNE WITH BEANS

Nutrition Facts
Serving Size 1 cup
Servings Per Container 2

Amount Per Serving About

Calories 290

Calories from Fat 60

Total Fat 7 grams

Saturated Fat 2.5 gram _

Cholesterol 35 mg

Sodium 940 mg -----look for a brand that has less sodium

Total Carbohydrate 38 grams

Dietary Fiber 13 grams

Sugars 3 grams

Protein 19 grams

VITAMIN A 20% **VITAMIN C** 0%
CALCIUM 10% **IRON** 20%

When shopping for chili or beans, look for the brand with the lowest sodium content. For example, Hormel Chili contains a whopping 1200 mg of sodium per serving.

S&W **GARBANZO BEANS**

("CECI BEANS" or "CHICK PEAS")

Nutrition Facts

Serving Size 1/2 cup

Amount Per Serving

Calories 80

Calories from Fat 15

Total Fat 1.5 grams

Saturated Fat 0 gram _

Sodium 460 mg

Cholesterol 0 mg

Total Carbohydrate 18 grams

Dietary Fiber 7 grams

Sugars 2 grams

Protein 6 grams

Vitamin A 0% **Vitamin C** 8% **Iron** 8% **Calcium** 6%

50% less sodium garbanzo beans have only 230 mg of sodium per serving.

_S&W_ KIDNEY BEAMS
PREMIUM DARK RED

Nutrition Facts
Serving Size 1/2_cup
Servings Per Container 2

Amount Per Serving

Calories 100

Calories from Fat 5

Total Fat 0.5 grams

Saturated Fat 0 gram _

Cholesterol 0 mg

Sodium 460 mg ------the 59%-less sodium can contains only 230 mg sodium per serving.

Total Carbohydrate 23 grams

Dietary Fiber 6 grams

Sugars 8 grams

Protein 7 grams

Along with "Top Ramen" I can't think of many foods that are nutritionally worse. The only ingredient missing is radioactivity. Ramen noodles are a common cause of afternoon school headaches. It is loaded with sodium and MSG. Hot dogs are another headache producer loaded with sodium and nitrites.

LUNCH

**MARUCHAN INSTANT LUNCH
RAMEN NOODLES
(CHICKEN FLAVOR)**

Nutrition Facts
Serving Size 1
Servings Per Container 1
Amount Per Serving
Calories 290
Calories from Fat 110
Total Fat 12 grams
Saturated Fat 6 gram
Cholesterol 3 mg
Sodium 1380 mg
Total Carbohydrate 37 grams
Dietary Fiber 2 grams
Sugars 2 grams
Protein 6 grams

By now you should be able to understand why lunchables are a poor choice. The fat and sodium content is enormous and only one gram of fiber! Leave this one out of your child's lunch box.

LUNCHABLES[144]
LEAN TURKEY BREAST; FUDGE SANDWICH COOKIE; AMERICAN CHEESE

Nutrition Facts
Serving Size 1 package
Servings Per Container 1
Amount Per Serving
Calories 370
Calories from Fat 180
Total Fat 20 grams
Saturated Fat 8 grams
Cholesterol 50 mg
Sodium 1390 mg
Total Carbohydrate 33 grams
Dietary Fiber 1 gram
Sugars 10 grams
Protein 16 grams

[145] Reduced-Fat Lunchables is a product made up of "98 % Fat Free" smoked turkey breast, cheddar cheese, and wheat crackers. Don't be fooled!!! It contains 9 grams of fat, 5 grams of which is saturated, plus a megadose of sodium at 1580 mg per serving. It also contains nitrite.

KRAFT MACARONI AND CHEESE

Serving size: ¼ cup------now what child or teenager eats only ¼ of a cup?

Amount per serving:

Calories 290---multiple that by 4 if the true portion is a cup

Calories from fat: 54

Total Fat: 6 grams

Saturated Fat: 3.5 grams or 14 grams for a full cup

Cholesterol: 20mg

Sodium: 590mg for ¼ cup or 2360mg for a full cup

Total Carbohydrate: 49 grams

Dietary Fiber 1 gram

Sugars: 0

Protein 28 grams

Barilla Plus Thin Spaghetti

Nutrition Facts
Serving Size: 100 grams
Calories: 370
Calories From Fat: 30
Total Fat: 3 grams
Saturated Fat 0.5 grams
Trans Fat 0
Cholesterol 0
Sodium 45 mg
Total Carbohydrate 67 grams
Dietary Fiber 7 grams
Sugars 3 grams
Protein 17 grams

DeCecco Spaghetti-100% Whole Wheat

Nutrition Facts
Serving Size: 2 oz
Calories 200
Calories from Fat 15
Total Fat 1.5 grams
Saturated Fat 0
Cholesterol - less than 5 mg
Sodium 0
Total Carbohydrate 39 grams
Dietary Fiber 5 grams
Sugars 1 gram
Protein 8 grams

Break the Monotony?

HORMEL SPAM

"In 1963, Spam was introduced to various private and public schools in South Florida as cheap food and even for art sculptures. Due to the success of the introduction, Hormel Foods also introduced school "color-themed" spam. The first being a blue and green variety which is still traditionally used in some private schools of South Florida."

Nutrition Facts

Serving size: 2 oz-listed but the usual serving is closer to 4 oz!!! so double all of the figures!!

Calories per serving:	174 X 2
Calories from fat:	137 X 2
Total Fat	15 grams X 2
Saturated Fat	6 grams X 2
Trans Fat:	0
Cholesterol	39 mg X 2
Sodium	767 mg X 2
Total Carbohydrate:	2 grams X 2
Dietary Fiber:	0
Sugars:	?
Protein	7 grams X 2

In Hawaii, Spam is so popular it is sometimes referred to as "The Hawaiian Steak". The primary ingredient is in Spam is chopped pork shoulder meat mixed with ham.

HEBREW NATIONAL HOT DOGS

(does not answer to a higher power)

Nutrition Facts

Serving Size 1 Frank

Amount Per Serving
Calories 150
Calories from Fat 126
Total Fat 14 grams
Saturated Fat 6 grams
Cholesterol 30 mg
Sodium 370 mg
Total Carbohydrate 1 gram
Dietary Fiber 0 grams
Sugars 0 grams
Protein 6 grams
CONTAINS SODIUM NITRITE

OSCAR MAYER WIENERS
(MADE WITH TURKEY AND PORK)

Nutrition Facts
Serving Size 1 Link
Servings Per Container 10

Amount Per Serving
Calories 140
Calories from Fat 120
Total Fat 13 grams
Saturated Fat 4.5 grams
Cholesterol 45 mg
Sodium 440 mg
Total Carbohydrate 1 gram
Dietary Fiber 0 grams
Sugars <1 gram
Protein 5 grams

Ingredients: Mechanically separated turkey, pork, water, salt, contains less than 2% corn syrup, dextrose, flavor, sodium phosphate, sodium erythrobate, sodium nitrite.
Do you still wish you were an Oscar Mayer Wiener?

CELESTE PIZZA FOR ONE
(WITH SAUSAGE, GREEN & RED PEPPERS, PEPPERONI, MUSH-ROOMS, ONIONS & OLIVES.)

Nutrition Facts
Serving Size 1 Pizza
Servings Per Container 1

Amount Per Serving
Calories 580
Calories from Fat 240
Total Fat 27 grams
Saturated Fat 9 grams
Cholesterol 25 mg
Sodium 1290 mg
Total Carbohydrate 49 grams
Dietary Fiber 6 grams
Sugars 6 grams
Protein 22 grams
VITAMIN A 25% **VIT C** 11% **CALCIUM** 40% **IRON** 15%

If your school lunch program offers pizza, get a copy of the Nutrition Facts from the provider. Beware of the dietician who defends pizza because it is high in calcium and protein. There are healthier ways to get these nutrients.

THE FOLLOWING NUTRITION FACTS ON TWO FROZEN HEALTHY CHOICE LUNCHES ARE EXAMPLES TO BE COMPARED WITH SWANSON HUNGRY-MAN FROZEN FRIED CHICKEN AND SAFEWAY CHICKEN POT PIE.

HEALTHY CHOICE

CHICKEN & VEGETABLES MARSALA

Nutrition Facts
Serving Size 1 Meal
Servings Per Container 1

Amount Per Serving

Calories 230

Calories from Fat 15

Total Fat 1.5 grams

Saturated Fat 0.5 grams

Polyunsaturated Fat 0.5 grams

Cholesterol 30 mg

Sodium 440 mg

Total Carbohydrate 32 grams

Dietary Fiber 3 grams

Sugars 1 gram

Protein 22 grams

VITAMIN A 10% **VITAMIN C** 6%
CALCIUM 6% **IRON** 10%

HEALTHY CHOICE

GINGER CHICKEN HUNAN

Nutrition Facts
Serving Size 1 Meal
Servings Per Container 1

Amount Per Serving

Calories 350

Calories from Fat 20

Total Fat 2.5 grams

Saturated Fat 0.5 grams

Polyunsaturated Fat 1 gram

Monounsaturated Fat 1 gram

Cholesterol 25 mg

Sodium 430 mg

Total Carbohydrate 59 grams

Dietary Fiber 5 grams

Sugars 11 grams –a little less than 3 teaspoons

Protein 24 grams

VITAMIN A 15% **VITAMIN C** 0%
CALCIUM 6% **IRON** 15%

SWANSON HUNGRY-MAN

FRIED CHICKEN, MASHED POTATO

CORN & APPLE-CRANBERRY CRUMB DES-SERT

Nutrition Facts
Serving Size 1 Package
Servings Per Container 1
Amount Per Serving
Calories 780
Calories from Fat 350
Total Fat 35 grams
Saturated Fat 12 grams !!!!!
Cholesterol 105 mg
Sodium 1700 mg !!!!!!!
Total Carbohydrate 74 grams
Dietary Fiber 8 grams
Sugars 15 grams- almost 4 teaspoons
Protein 33 grams

SAFEWAY HOME STYLE "MAIN DISH"

OVEN BAKED
CHICKEN POT PIE

Nutrition Facts
Serving Size 7 oz.
Servings Per Container 4

Amount Per Serving
Calories 530
Calories from Fat 280
Total Fat 31 grams
Saturated Fat 11 grams
Trans Fat 1.5 mg
Cholesterol 30 mg
Sodium 800 mg
Total Carbohydrate 44 grams
Dietary Fiber 3 grams
Soluble Fiber
Insoluble Fiber
Sugars 6 grams
Protein 14 gram
VITAMIN A 25% **CALCIUM** 6%

SNACKS

The single largest source of fat among people who eat high-fat diets is french fries. Hamburgers are second. Buy the leanest meat to make your hamburgers and stay clear of the Big Mac or the many other super-charged hamburger combinations. Check those "baked" French fries for fat content. Try those vegetarian burgers, such as wholesome hearty foods burgers, morningstar farms garden vege and garden grain patties, fantastic foods nature's burger or boca burgers. They have little fat, good taste, and are enjoyed by most children when served on a fresh bun with ketchup, non-fat or reduced fat mayo, or fresh salsa. Parents are always looking for a special treat to put in their child's lunch box. Fresh fruit is always a safe choice. Before buying a treat, check the nutrition label. Here are a couple of suggestions.

Don't be fooled. Low fat almost always means high sugar!

ENTENMANN'S *LIGHT* FAT FREE BROWNIES

Nutrition Facts
Serving Size 1/10 Strip
Servings Per Container 10

Amount Per Serving

Calories 120

Calories from Fat 0

Total Fat 0 grams

Saturated Fat 0 grams

Cholesterol 0 mg

Sodium 125 mg

Total Carbohydrate 27 grams

Dietary Fiber 1 gram

Sugars 20 grams!!!!!!!!!!!

Protein 2 grams

SARA LEE FAT FREE ANGEL FOOD CAKE
(HIGH SUGAR)

Nutrition Facts
Serving Size 1/5 Cake
Servings Per Container 5

Amount Per Serving

Calories 180

Calories from Fat 0

Total Fat 0 grams

Saturated Fat 0 grams _

Cholesterol 0 mg

Sodium 285 mg

Total Carbohydrate 43 grams

Dietary Fiber 1 gram

Sugars 24 grams___(6 teaspoons sugar)

Protein 3 grams

HERSHEY'S Chocolate SYRUP

Nutrition Facts
Serving Size 2 Tbs.
Servings Per Container 11

Amount Per Serving

Calories 0

Calories from Fat

Total Fat 0 grams

Saturated Fat 0 grams

Cholesterol 0 mg

Sodium 35 mg

Total Carbohydrate 27 grams

Dietary Fiber 0 grams

Sugars 22 grams---OVER 5 teaspoons per serving---on top of high sugar and fat ice cream.

Protein <1 gram

COMPARE THIS WITH HERSHEY'S SYRUP-LITE

Servings Size: 2 Tbsp.	45 Calories
Calories from fat 0	
Sugars 10 grams	

▲ ▲ ▲

"What shall I feed my child?" is on the mind of every parent. I am grateful to the many people who helped me answer this question. My wife, Linda, deserves special recognition for encouraging me to update my year 2000 edition of Feed Your Child Right From Birth through Teens. Linda is an OB-Gyn Nurse Practitioner and has a first hand understanding of the confusion most parents have sorting through the trees of nutritional information from disinformation and myth. Her critical review of each page kept me focused. Dr. Paul Steinman, a highly respected pediatrician in Marin County, California was helpful in reviewing this book,. I am especially thankful to Mary Greenberg for her diligence and editing skill. Once again I am grateful to my original publisher, M. Evans and Company, Inc., for recognizing the importance of this book. Thanks to Jenny Legun Chandler, Senior Publishing Consultant at CreateSpace, an Amazon company, and Team Synergy, this book is now updated and will be available in Paperback and on Amazon Kindle.

▲ ▲ ▲

THE MARIN COUNTY DIET
FEED YOUR CHILD RIGHT FROM BIRTH

F

G

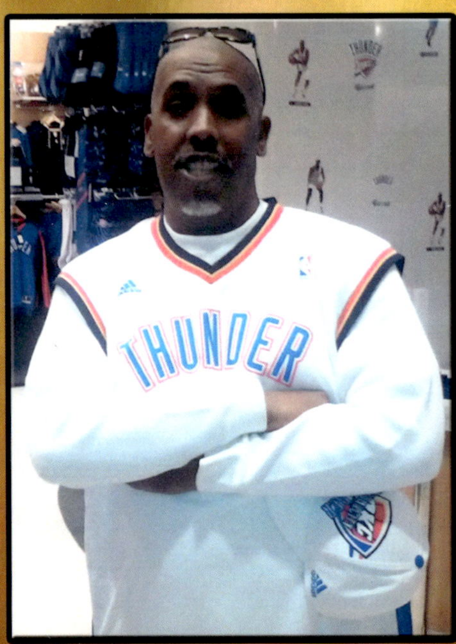

About The Author

Burning The Candle at Both Ends is Bryce Turner's sophomore book project his freshman book was "Off The Front Line".

Bryce spends most of his time speaking to the youth and the less fortunate, giving them positive advice, along with hope and inspiration to push forward in life, despite of their situations.

He is also involved with the family business helping out doing Interior Restoration, whenever he is not in the lab working on his next book project.

Bryce is in transition toward getting out of the worldly things in life, and focusing more on serving Jehovah, and doing his will one day in the near future.

He is one of OKC Thunder biggest fans, hoping they win their first Championship in 2014!

$19.95

www.ingramcontent.com/pod-product-compliance
Lightning Source LLC
Chambersburg PA
CBHW060235100426
42742CB00011B/1540

* 9 7 8 0 6 1 5 7 8 9 2 9 3 *